the bipolar workbook

the bipolar workbook

Tools for Controlling Your Mood Swings

Monica Ramirez Basco, PhD

THE GUILFORD PRESS
New York   London

© 2006 The Guilford Press
A Division of Guilford Publications, Inc.
72 Spring Street, New York, NY 10012
www.guilford.com

Printed in the United States of America

This book is printed on acid-free paper.

Last digit is print number: 9 8 7 6 5 4 3 2

Library of Congress Cataloging-in-Publication Data

Basco, Monica Ramirez.
   The bipolar workbook : tools for controlling your mood swings /
Monica Ramirez Basco.
        p.   cm.
   Includes bibliographical references and index.
   ISBN-10: 1-59385-162-6; ISBN-13: 978-1-59385-162-0 (alk. paper)
   1. Manic–depressive illness—Popular works. 2. Manic–
depressive illness—Treatment—Popular works. 3. Manic–depressive
illness—Treatment—Problems, exercises, etc.   I. Title.
   RC516.B356 2006
   616.89′506—dc22
                                                    2005014041

Contents

Test Your Knowledge of Bipolar Disorder

Circle *true* or *false*. The correct answers are on pages viii–x.

True or False   1. Bipolar disorder can cause both depression and mania.

True or False   2. You can be depressed and manic at the same time.

True or False   3. Medications are necessary to control the symptoms of bipolar disorder.

True or False   4. All you need to do to stay well is take your medication every day.

True or False   5. There is nothing you can do to stop depression or mania once it starts.

True or False   6. Sleep loss can trigger a manic episode.

True or False   7. To cope with bipolar disorder, you have to give up the exciting parts of life.

True or False   8. Having the illness usually means giving up your career goals.

True or False   9. You can handle this illness on your own. You don't need help.

True or False   10. You don't have bipolar disorder. The doctors are wrong.

Test Answers

1. Bipolar disorder can cause both depression and mania.

TRUE. Most people who have bipolar disorder have episodes of depression and mania throughout their lives. Some may have more depression. Some may have more episodes of mania. Everyone's symptoms are a little different. To learn more about your pattern of symptoms, read Chapters 3 and 4.

2. You can be depressed and manic at the same time.

TRUE. This is called a *mixed episode*. During mixed episodes people can feel wound up, have racing thoughts and difficulty sitting still, as in mania, but feel down, hopeless, and suicidal, as in depression. Mixed states can also alternate quickly between depression and mania, each lasting only hours or a few days. They can be difficult to diagnose because they do not look like typical episodes of depression or mania. Learn more about how diagnoses are made in Chapter 2.

3. Medications are necessary to control the symptoms of bipolar disorder

TRUE. Although many people prefer to "tough out" periods of depression and mania without medications, it's clear that control of the illness and prevention of future relapses depend on effective medication management. Most people prefer not to take medications and, in fact, have a lot of trouble sticking with a medication regimen for long periods of time. Chapter 6 has some ideas for dealing with medication.

4. All you need to do to stay well is take your medication every day.

FALSE. There's a lot more to managing bipolar disorder than taking medication. Unfortunately, even when people take their medications very consistently, other things like stress, illness, or change of season can cause symptoms to return. When symptoms return, most people don't function well at work, with their families, or with their friends. Medication can help to control the symptoms, but it doesn't fix the problems at work or home. Special symptom and life management skills are needed to fill in the gaps where medication does not do the trick. Chapter 1 provides an overview of the things you can do to help control your illness and solve problems of daily life.

5. There is nothing you can do to stop depression or mania once it starts.

FALSE. In addition to taking medication, there are a number of things you can do to help control the symptoms of depression and mania. Chapters 4 through 10 will cover methods you can use to change your actions and thoughts in a way that controls manic and depressive symptoms. You will also learn ways to come to terms with the illness and manage your life to reduce the chance of recurrence.

6. Sleep loss can trigger a manic episode.

TRUE. Losing consistent nighttime sleep puts people at risk for becoming manic. People who have bipolar disorder tend to be night people more than morning people. However, staying up later than usual and getting less sleep seems to spur a manic episode or make it worse once mania has begun. Chapter 5 offers methods for improving the consistency of sleep, as well as things you can do to overcome fatigue and lethargy caused by sleep loss.

7. To cope with bipolar disorder, you have to give up the exciting parts of life.

FALSE. It's a common misconception that you have to live a quiet and unexciting life, with restrictions on activity, work, and play, to control the illness. This is rarely the case. Living with bipolar disorder does mean exercising some moderation, however. The methods in Chapter 4 for learning when your symptoms are worsening will help you know when to slow down and when to ask for help. Strategies presented throughout the workbook will help you keep your symptoms in check. And the techniques in Chapters 5, 9, and 10 for managing stress, making decisions, and setting reasonable limits will help you live a happy and productive life and minimize intrusions caused by the illness.

8. Having the illness usually means giving up your career goals.

FALSE. Many vibrant and successful people have bipolar disorder. They have figured out how to work with the illness and still accomplish their goals. Numerous exercises are provided in this workbook to help you feel in control of your illness rather than feeling like it controls you. It requires a lot of work, more than just taking medication every day. But if you're determined to succeed, the illness does not have to get in the way.

9. You can handle this illness on your own. You don't need help.

FALSE. Everyone needs support, especially when struggling with a serious illness. Support can come from family, friends, work associates, self-help groups like Alcoholics Anonymous and the Depression and Bipolar Support Alliance, Internet support groups, and health care providers. Isolation from others usually makes matters worse. You might avoid the stress that can come from social contact, but you also will miss out on the benefits of having people to talk to, to help in times of crisis, to love you and convince you of your worth, and to give you a reason to live. If you are having problems getting along with others, look over Chapter 9 for some tips.

10. You don't have bipolar disorder. The doctors are wrong.

MAYBE. If you're reading this book, you or someone close to you thinks you have bipolar disorder. However, diagnoses are sometimes difficult to make, especially if you're young or you've struggled with substance abuse or alcohol problems. The information provided in Chapters 1, 2, and 3 will help you decide whether you have the illness. If you fit the bill, but are not ready to deal with it, skip to Chapter 7 to help you work toward acceptance of the diagnosis.

chapter one

Taking Control of Your Illness

In this chapter you will:

✓ Read about the four steps to controlling depression and mania.
✓ Find out why medications alone don't control your illness.
✓ Learn how your reactions to your symptoms can help you or hurt you.
✓ Discover how this workbook will help you take control of your symptoms.

This workbook is designed to guide you through the process of learning what you can do, in addition to taking medication regularly, to control your symptoms of bipolar disorder. There is a lot you can accomplish. You can learn to lessen and avoid symptoms of depression, mania, hypomania, irritability, and anxiety, as well as cope with the many ways your illness can interfere with your life. You can use this book on your own, make it part of your individual or group therapy, or work through it with your psychiatrist. Each chapter offers information, skills, and exercises that can help you learn to cope with your emotions, control negative thinking, minimize physical symptoms, deal with medication issues, manage problems of daily life, and generally come to terms with having bipolar disorder.

If you commit the time to practice and learn each method, the exercises in this workbook can help you learn the facts about bipolar disorder, achieve more stability, discover new ways to keep the symptoms from coming back, get more out of treatment, and reach your goals in life.

How Can You Control the Illness?

Bipolar disorder is biological in nature, but it causes both physical and psychological symptoms. The physical symptoms include impairments in sleep, energy, appetite, and concentration. The psychological symptoms include changes in thoughts, feelings, and choice of actions. This workbook will provide you with a host of tools to control your mood swings and to improve the quality of your life by managing the physical and psychological symptoms of depression and mania.

The overall goal of this workbook is to help you prevent recurrences of depression and mania. To accomplish this you will need to learn two important things:

1. **How to recognize the early warning signs that the physical and psychological symptoms of bipolar disorder are returning.**
2. **How to act quickly to stop the symptoms before they become severe. That means taking action to control symptoms before they become full episodes of depression and mania by correcting and controlling the thinking problems, activity changes, and emotional upsets caused by the illness.**

The interventions throughout the workbook are geared toward helping you in four ways—to see symptoms coming, take precautions, reduce your symptoms, and check your progress. The outline below summarizes the steps you can take to control your mood swings.

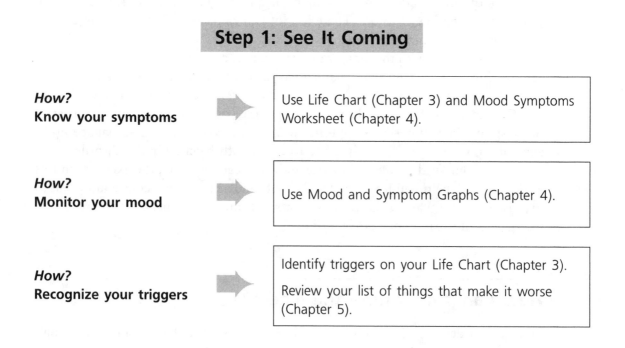

Step 1: See It Coming

How?
Know your symptoms ➡ Use Life Chart (Chapter 3) and Mood Symptoms Worksheet (Chapter 4).

How?
Monitor your mood ➡ Use Mood and Symptom Graphs (Chapter 4).

How?
Recognize your triggers ➡ Identify triggers on your Life Chart (Chapter 3).

Review your list of things that make it worse (Chapter 5).

Step 2: Take Precautions

How?
Don't make it worse

➡

Learn to get enough sleep (Chapter 5).

Stick with medications (Chapter 6).

Avoid symptom triggers (Chapters 5 and 6).

How?
Add positives

➡

Learn to strengthen relationships (Chapters 5 and 8).

Set personal goals (Chapter 6).

Work toward adjustment to the illness (Chapter 7).

Develop healthy habits (Chapter 5).

How?
Decrease negatives

➡

Solve problems (Chapters 5 and 8).

Control worry and rumination (Chapter 5).

Avoid overstimulation (Chapters 5 and 9).

Step 3: Reduce Your Symptoms

How?
Stop inactivity

➡

Use Activity Schedule.

Break it down and take it on, and use "A" list/"B" list (Chapter 5).

How?
Change your thinking

➡

Use the *catch it, control it, correct it* methods (Chapters 8 and 9).

How?
Reverse mental meltdown

➡

Use the *slow it, focus it, structure it* methods (Chapter 10).

How?
Reduce hyperactivity

➡

Control overstimulation.

Keep desire for change in check.

Set limits on activity with goal setting.

Get some sleep (Chapter 5).

Step 4: Check Your Progress

How?
Monitor your mood and symptom changes

Use Mood Graphs (Chapter 4).

Use Mood Symptoms Worksheet (Chapter 4).

Get feedback from others (Chapter 9).

Why It Takes More Than Medication

Medications that effectively control symptoms of depression and mania, mood swings, anxiety, irritability, and sleep problems are the cornerstone of managing illnesses like bipolar disorder. Bipolar disorder is a biological illness that causes changes in the way your brain processes the chemicals your body naturally produces. Medications are designed to correct this problem by providing these chemicals or neurotransmitters when they are lacking or by helping your brain use them more efficiently. Without medication, psychological approaches like those presented in this workbook may be only minimally effective. But even with medication, you, like most people with bipolar disorder, will probably need more to gain the greatest possible control over your symptoms and to prevent relapse.

• You need backup interventions for those times when you don't take your medications consistently or when they are not working fully. Most people with bipolar disorder have trouble taking medication on a regular basis, especially when their symptoms have improved or when side effects are unpleasant.

• You need ways to minimize stress, cope with changes of season, and avoid sleep loss—all factors that can cause symptoms to return even when you take medication every day.

• You need healthy and effective ways to control your symptoms instead of giving in to the temptation to use alcohol or street drugs to help you sleep, calm your nerves, or change your mood. Alcohol and street drugs are not usually safe to use when you are taking psychiatric medications, and they can interfere with the potency of some medications.

• You need methods for examining and managing your lifestyle so that it doesn't lead to sleep loss, poor eating habits, or unhealthy behaviors that can increase the risk of relapse.

• You may find yourself going through times when part of you rejects the idea of having this illness, does not want to take medications, or is unwilling to make the modifications to your lifestyle that might help reduce or eliminate symptoms. At the same time another part of you knows what you should do to take care of yourself. You need some strategies for sorting out your feelings about the illness and the treatment when you feel conflicted about it.

- Depression and mania can make it hard to organize your thoughts, make decisions, and solve problems. You need ways to reverse the mental meltdown that makes it hard to think.

- Medications may remove symptoms, but if you've had financial, legal, or family problems as a result of bipolar disorder, you'll be left with those problems even when your symptoms have improved. You need ways to resolve the problems that stress you so that you can improve the quality of your life.

Fortunately, there are methods you can learn to fill the gaps that medication treatment leaves. Strategies for controlling symptoms, preventing relapse, and solving problems are explained in this workbook. Mastering these strategies will help you come to terms with your illness, give you a reason to stick with medication treatment, and keep the ups and downs from interfering with your life.

The Ups and Downs of Bipolar Disorder

Many different things can trigger depression and mania in people who have bipolar disorder, but sometimes they occur for no specific reason at all. Once an episode starts, however, your reaction to it can make symptoms better or worse. This is why.

Depression or mania will cause **changes in your thought processes and your emotions,** as shown in the diagram. Your thoughts—what you think about and how you think—are also referred to as *cognitions*. Fill out Worksheet 1.1 to remind yourself of the emotions and cognitions you've experienced during periods of depression and mania.

Changes in your emotions and thought processes **affect behavior.** They can **color the types of actions** you choose to take, such as staying out late to have fun because you feel terrific and don't want the day to end, starting a new project because you're full of new ideas, or avoiding interactions with others because you're feeling bad about yourself and don't

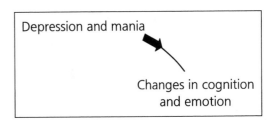

Depression and mania affect thoughts and feelings.

| worksheet 1.1 | **Cognitions and Emotions** |

Emotions	Cognitions
Emotional changes are feelings like sadness, despair, and anxiety and feeling high, euphoric, or irritable. These emotions are usually intense and will last for days, weeks, or months at a time. They are not just reactions to exciting or upsetting events.	Both the content and the process of your thinking can change during episodes of depression and mania. Content changes are what you think about. For example, when depressed you have more negative thoughts and when manic you might have new and exciting ideas. The thought processes that change are the speed of your thinking, how well you can concentrate, the clarity of your thoughts, and your decision-making ability.
Circle the words that describe your emotions during depression or mania. sad empty blue lonely worried anxious tense uptight irritable annoyed angry euphoric elevated high happy ecstatic	*Circle the words that describe your cognitive changes during depression or mania.* **Process changes:** slow confused forgetful poor judgment indecisive muddled unrealistic foggy creative racing **Content changes:** negative hopeless self-critical paranoid new plans optimistic

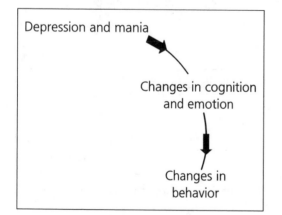

Thoughts and feelings affect behavior.

want others to see you depressed. In the following exercise (Worksheet 1.2), try to match the emotions, thoughts, and actions that might go together during episodes of depression and mania.

The **quality of your actions can change** when you are depressed or manic. You might be more disorganized or jump from one activity to another when manic. You might move more slowly than usual when depressed.

It does not take long before **changes in**

worksheet 1.2	**Moods, Thoughts, and Actions**

Mood	Thoughts	Actions
Sad	*I have the best idea ever.*	Decides not to go to party.
Nervous	*There is nothing I can do about my problem.*	Snaps at a friend.
Euphoric	*He's getting on my nerves.*	Gives up.
Irritable	*I'll freeze up and not know what to say.*	Leaves work early to start a new project.

From *The Bipolar Workbook* by Monica Ramirez Basco. Copyright 2006 by The Guilford Press. Permission to photocopy this form is granted to purchasers of this book for personal use only (see copyright page for details).

types and quality of behavior affect your ability to function effectively at home, work, or in social situations, as shown in the diagram. Here are some examples.

- Taking action before thinking things through can lead to errors in judgment or poor decision making.
- Slowness in movement and fatigue can interfere with fulfilling obligations.
- Giving up means that problems may not get solved.
- Starting too many projects means nothing gets finished.
- Leaving work early because you're tired may lead to reprimands from the boss.
- Avoiding people means missing out on fun.
- Snapping at people may start conflict and damage relationships.

When your functioning declines and you're unable to compensate for it, **problems often develop.**

For example, poor job performance can lead to termination of employment. Failing to meet responsibilities at home can cause conflict with your parents or spouse, strain marriages, or interfere with family

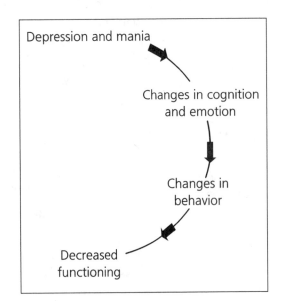

Behavior changes affect functioning.

Answers for Worksheet 1.2

Mood	Thoughts	Actions
Sad	*I have the best idea ever.*	Decides not to go to party.
Nervous	*There is nothing I can do about my problem.*	Snaps at a friend.
Euphoric	*He's getting on my nerves.*	Gives up.
Irritable	*I'll freeze up and not know what to say.*	Leaves work early to start a new project.

communication. Impulsivity and poor decision making can lead to financial problems and relationship problems. Typical problems are shown in the table on page 9.

What problems have you experienced in your life that you think might be attributable to having bipolar disorder? These could be problems caused by the symptoms of the disorder as described above, or they could have been caused indirectly when mania and depression kept you from dealing with everyday life issues. On Worksheet 1.3, make some notes on the types of problems you think you might have had in your life because of bipolar disorder. This list will help you gain control of your symptoms in two ways. One, if you see old problems coming back, it may be a sign that it is time to take action to control your symptoms. Two, if you focus on skills that help you prevent new problems from forming, you can reduce the stress that can cause a relapse.

Having to cope with problems will cause stress for anyone, but because you have bipolar disorder the risks are greater for you. Nighttime worry about problems can in-

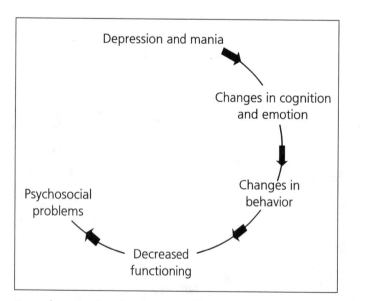

Poor functioning leads to problems.

Problems Caused by Poor Functioning

Changes in functioning	Possible problems
Acting without thinking and poor decision making	Quitting a job without having a new one when you can't afford it
Not fulfilling role obligations	Neglecting children's well-being
Spending excessively, not paying bills	Eviction from home, repossession of belongings
Arguing with people at work instead of solving problems calmly	Termination of employment
Drinking excessively or using street drugs	Legal problems, health problems, family problems

---

worksheet 1.3 | **Problems Associated with Having Bipolar Disorder**

Relationship problems:

Work problems:

School problems:

Legal problems:

Financial problems:

Family problems:

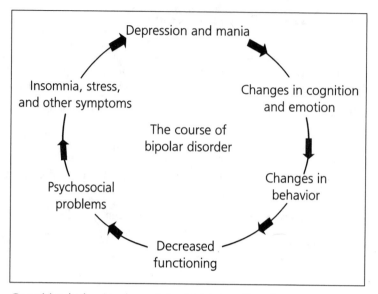

Depression and mania

Insomnia, stress,
and other symptoms

Changes in cognition
and emotion

The course of
bipolar disorder

Psychosocial
problems

Changes in
behavior

Decreased
functioning

Cognitive-behavioral model of bipolar disorder.

terfere with sleep, and sleep loss can induce mania. Attempting to relieve stress with alcohol can make depression worse and can also interfere with sleep. Fatigue from sleep loss can cause further decline in work performance, can lower motivation to handle problems, and may lead you to give up and give in to depression. **All of this can worsen symptoms of depression and mania, and the cycle perpetuates itself.**

Cognitive-Behavioral Therapy for Bipolar Disorder

This description may make the cycle of symptoms and problems in bipolar disorder seem overwhelming and impossible to control, but in fact it's possible to learn effective ways to manage your illness. This workbook provides you with the tools for controlling your mood swings that are usually taught in cognitive-behavioral therapy, or CBT. CBT is a skills-oriented type of psychotherapy that teaches you ways to straighten out problems in thinking, control your emotions, and cope more effectively with your symptoms and your life problems. Throughout this workbook, you will be provided with the tools that cognitive-behavioral therapists use to help people cope with depression and mania. Here is how it works.

The overall plan is for you get to know yourself and your pattern of symptoms well enough to know when they are coming back and to learn CBT skills for managing them. The end result is that if you do all that you can to control symptoms and work closely with your doctor to find the right medications, you will have shorter times of illness and longer times of wellness.

Throughout this workbook you will learn ways to break the cycle of depression and mania with tools that control symptoms at each point in the sequence. First you have to learn to recognize where you are in the cycle of changes in thoughts, emotions, actions, and functioning. This will be accomplished by developing an early warning system, using the methods described in Chapters 3 and 4. Next, you will need to learn ways to control the mood swings and changes in thinking that seem to come early in the course of depression and mania. This can be accomplished by learning the methods in Chapters 8 and 9 for evaluating your thoughts and removing any distortions in your thinking. When you do this, your depressed, euphoric, and irritable moods will usually decrease in intensity. In Chapter 10 you will learn to slow down and sort through your thoughts in a more systematic way so that you can make good decisions and cope more effectively with the changes you're experiencing. When you are able to do this, you will usually feel less anxious, irritated, and overwhelmed. Taken together, the methods used to control your cognitive and emotional changes in depression and mania will help to break the cycle. The mental and emotional symptoms will lessen, and they will be less likely to negatively affect your behavior.

Another way to break the cycle of bipolar disorder is to control the behaviors that may be making symptoms worse. That includes staying up all night, drinking too much, avoiding people, or procrastinating in solving problems. In Chapter 5 you'll learn several different strategies for coping more effectively, taking positive action, solving problems, keeping yourself from getting out of control, and breaking out of procrastination and lethargy. When you change your actions, you will think better of yourself and feel more hopeful about your ability to cope. Changing behavior helps to improve the cognitive and emotional symptoms of depression and mania. The reverse is also true. When your mood and attitude are better, you will engage in more productive behaviors.

If you realize you are in the middle of a cycle of depression or mania only after your thoughts, feelings, and actions have changed for the worse, you can learn to work your way out of the episode by taking your medications more consistently and by taking steps to avoid aggravating the situation. The CBT methods covered in Chapters 5 and 6 will help you get back on track when you feel out of control and when you are having trouble taking the medication your doctor has prescribed. If you can get back into the swing of things, you can regain control over your thoughts, feelings, and actions.

You might find that the way you've behaved during periods of depression or mania has caused new problems or has brought more stress into your life. Having too much stress worsens your mood, interferes with your sleep, and keeps depression and mania going. To break the cycle, you will need to learn the stress management strategies covered in Chapters 5 and 10. They will help you resolve your difficulties so you can lessen your worry and get a good night's sleep.

When combined with effective medication management, these cognitive-behavioral strategies can help you take control of your illness so that you can reach your goals and have a happy and productive life.

How to Use This Workbook

This workbook was written for four types of readers. The first type is someone who was diagnosed recently and doesn't yet know a great deal about how to manage his or her illness. **Goals for the newly diagnosed are to:**

1. Better understand your illness.
2. Learn ways to make treatment work.
3. Find out how to live with and manage your symptoms.

The second type of person this workbook is suited for has struggled with bipolar disorder for some time and doesn't feel he or she has achieved stability. **Goals for the experienced person who is still working toward greater stability are to:**

1. Get more out of medication treatment.
2. Learn skills to control your mood swings.
3. Gain acceptance of your illness and treatment.

The third type of person with bipolar disorder who is the focus of this book has found a medication regimen that works and wants to learn more about how to maintain stability. **Goals to help this person maintain stability are to:**

1. Know your vulnerabilities.
2. Prevent relapse.
3. Strengthen relationships.
4. Find purpose in life.

The fourth type of reader is the family member of someone who has bipolar disorder who wants to learn what he or she can do to help. Those individuals can be supportive, offer assistance, or help remind the person with the illness to use the methods learned. **Goals for the family member are to:**

1. **Try to understand the nature of bipolar disorder.**
2. **Know the signs of symptoms returning.**
3. **Learn how to encourage treatment and not interfere with it.**

If you fall into one of these four groups, you can work through this book from beginning to end or skip ahead to the sections of the workbook that pertain to you. Another way to use this workbook is to look over the table on pages 14–15 and choose the areas that apply to you. Read those sections before you read the others.

This workbook is organized so you can start with general information about bipolar disorder in Chapters 1 and 2 and then begin to put together your own personal history of symptoms and treatment. The exercises in Chapters 3 and 4 will help you develop your own early warning system so that you can identify recurrences of depression, mania, hypomania, or mixed states as soon as they begin. This will give you a head start in taking action to stop the symptoms from progressing.

Beginning with Chapter 5 and throughout the remainder of the workbook, you will be provided with methods for preventing and controlling symptoms of depression and mania. Chapter 6 helps you get the most out of your medication treatment, and Chapter 7 will help you out if you're having difficulty accepting the diagnosis of bipolar disorder and all that coping with the illness means. Chapters 8 and 9 will offer strategies for fighting off negative thinking and for keeping manic thinking from getting you into trouble. Chapter 10 will help you cope with poor concentration, difficulty organizing your thoughts, decision making, and mental overstimulation.

Illustrations: How It Works for Others with Bipolar Disorder

Throughout the workbook you'll find examples of how other people with bipolar disorder have responded to the exercises and interventions presented. They represent the first three types of readers described earlier. Tommy is 21 years old and was diagnosed with bipolar disorder only recently, so he is a good example of the first group. Amanda is 32 years old and has had bipolar disorder for several years but has not yet found a way to manage the symptoms. She would fall into the second group. Paul is 23 years old and was diagnosed with bipolar disorder as a child. He has worked closely with his psychiatrist for many years and has a pretty good regimen for controlling his symptoms most of the time. Raquel is 45 years old and has had the most experience with the illness. She has been through the adjustments that the others are just beginning to make, has come to terms with having bipolar disor-

Where Do I Start?

Understanding bipolar disorder

Do you need more information about the nature of bipolar disorder and its treatment? — Read Chapters 1 and 2.

Are you having trouble coming to terms with having bipolar disorder? — Read Chapters 2, 4, and 7.

Are you angry about having the illness and having to take medications? — Read Chapters 6 and 7.

Are you depressed about having bipolar disorder? — Read Chapters 7, 8, and 9.

Symptom awareness

Are you aware of the factors that influence your mood swings? — Read Chapter 4.

Do you think you are aware of your unique symptoms of depression, mania, hypomania, and mixed states? — Read Chapters 3 and 4.

Are you sometimes uncertain about whether your symptoms are returning? — Read Chapter 4.

Do you sometimes do things that make your mood or symptoms worse? — Read Chapters 4 and 5.

Coping with life

Is your sleep irregular? — Read Chapter 5.

Are you overstimulated by noise, people, or too much activity? — Read Chapter 5.

Medication treatment issues

Are you having difficulty taking medications on a daily basis? — Read Chapter 6.

Do you ever forget to take medications or decide you just don't want to take them? — Read Chapters 6 and 7.

Negative thinking

Are you overly negative, self-critical, or pessimistic? — Read Chapters 8 and 9.

Is it easy for you to see your failures and difficult to see your strengths? — Read Chapters 8 and 9.

Do other people think you take too many risks? Do you have trouble seeing it at the time, but realize it later? — Read Chapters 8 and 9.

Do you jump to conclusions or make assumptions that later turn out not to be true? — Read Chapters 8 and 9.

Where Do I Start? *(cont.)*

Mental clarity and concentration

Do you have any difficulty concentrating? Do you get distracted easily?	Read Chapter 10.
Are you disorganized?	Read Chapter 10.
Do you have trouble making decisions?	Read Chapter 10.

People problems

Are you isolated from others?	Read Chapter 5.
Do you have trouble solving problems with people?	Read Chapter 10.
Do people upset you?	Read Chapters 8 and 9.

Stress management

Is it hard to slow your mind and relax your body?	Read Chapters 5 and 10.
Are you easily overwhelmed with tasks and unable to take action?	Read Chapters 5 and 10.

der, and feels stable most of the time. Raquel and Paul fall into the third group of readers, those who have achieved relative stability. Having a feel for what each of these people has gone through and how they have used the methods in this book will help you know how their experiences might apply to you as you work through the exercises.

Tommy is a struggling college student. He has had two episodes of mania so far. The first episode was mild and did not last very long. He was diagnosed with bipolar disorder after his second episode because his symptoms were bad enough to require hospitalization. He was brought into the emergency room by police when he crashed his car into a light pole. His strange behavior made the police think he had been taking drugs along with the alcohol he had in the car. In the emergency room the doctor figured out that Tommy was actually manic. Tommy was not very cooperative in the hospital, and with the help of his parents, who thought his problem was drinking and nothing more, Tommy was discharged without medication. Unfortunately, he only got worse. The following week, Tommy's parents arranged through their family doctor to have him admitted to a psychiatric hospital because he was "talking crazy" about being a disciple of God and seeing angels flying around his room. He was started on a mood-stabilizing medication in the hospital, as well as an antipsychotic drug. He was more like his old self after a few weeks but did not really understand what had happened to him. Throughout the workbook, examples of Tommy's efforts to work through the exercises will be provided.

Like most people who have been diagnosed recently, Tommy knew very little about bipolar disorder, but he was pretty certain that he did not have it. He picked up the book from time to time and read through sections that caught his eye but did not really work through the entire program right away. His psychiatrist encouraged him to read more and learn about what he could do to control his symptoms. Tommy read the first few chapters, about the illness, but was not ready to buy into the idea that he had bipolar disorder. His mom was very worried about Tommy and frustrated by his lack of effort to educate himself. She read through the workbook as well as many other books on bipolar disorder so she would understand what was happening to her son. She encouraged Tommy to read Chapter 7, on the topic of denial, and to talk it over with her and with his doctor. After reading it Tommy was still not entirely convinced that he had bipolar disorder because he had not had enough experiences with the illness. On the other hand, he did not want to go to the hospital again, so he agreed to read the workbook a little at a time. Some of the exercises didn't seem to pertain to him, because he had not yet had a severe period of depression, but he recognized the symptoms of mania listed in Chapters 3 and 4 and made some effort to follow the guidelines in Chapter 5 for preventing them from returning. Tommy used the workbook like a reference book. Each time he had new experiences that might be related to bipolar disorder, he tried to find an exercise related to it. He would read through his old notes in the workbook and add new insights. Some of his notes are included in the workbook to show how someone newly diagnosed with bipolar disorder might approach the tasks.

Amanda is a good example of someone who has dealt with the many ups and downs of bipolar disorder but does not feel able to control it. A 32-year-old nurse who had her first episode of major depression in high school and her first manic episode in nursing school about 6 years ago, she has had other periods of depression, mania, and hypomania and has been under the care of a psychiatrist off and on over many years. In addition, Amanda has had supportive counseling to cope with periods of low mood. She knows she has bipolar disorder and wants to do what she can to control it for the sake of her family. She gets extremely irritated with her husband when she is manic, which has taken a toll on her marriage. She suffers from low-level depression much of the time and often has difficulty keeping her home clean and organized, doing her job at the hospital, and caring for her 5-year-old daughter. She has lost jobs for poor attendance when she was depressed and has walked off of jobs because her irritability and impulsiveness during manic spells have gotten the best of her.

Amanda picked up this workbook after a period of depression that really frightened her. She caught herself thinking that life was not worth living and that there was no hope for a better future. This was not Amanda's usual attitude, and when she came out of the depression, it greatly upset her that she had allowed her thinking to get so distorted. She kept thinking, "What if I had acted on those ideas?" Amanda was ready to work diligently through all the exercises in the workbook. She recognized her symptoms from the examples in Chapters 3 and 4 and knew she had coped poorly with them in the past. She made the adjustments in her lifestyle and in her reactions recommended in Chapter 5. Amanda was particularly interested in learning to control her distorted thinking, so she slowly and carefully worked through each exercise in Chapters 8, 9, and 10. She had worked through her denial about having the illness years ago but needed some help in taking her medications more consistently. She wanted treatment to work, but side effects and other problems always seemed to get in the way. Amanda used the methods in Chapter 6 to find a way to be more consistent with taking her medication. She was tired of all the ups and downs in her life, and each time she learned a new exercise for dealing with her distorted thoughts, her behavior changes, and her mood swings she felt like she had more control over her illness and her life. Amanda's examples are included throughout the workbook. If you think you're like Amanda, pay particular attention to how she completed each exercise.

Paul and Raquel are both good examples of people who have learned a great deal about how to manage bipolar disorder. Both have had bad experiences with depression and did not want to go there again. Paul is only 23 years old, but his bipolar disorder started during his elementary school years and he has been through enough treatment to be an expert on the issue. He did not go through a period of denial like Tommy had, because his parents explained to him when he was a young child what illness he had and how medication would help. He learned early in life that he felt better with medication than without it and that things went better at school and with his friends when he was more stable. Although Paul knew a great deal about the biology of bipolar disorder and was pretty consistent with taking medications, he did not know much about how his reactions contributed to his symptoms. He wanted to learn what he could do to keep his symptoms from flaring up without always having to take additional medications, which had been his strategy in the past. Paul only skimmed through the first three chapters because he had already read so much about the illness, as had his parents. He did not think he needed Chapters 6 and 7, because he had already accepted his illness and took his medication fairly consistently. What he wanted to learn were the methods in Chapter 5 for making himself less vulnerable to relapse by controlling his actions and the strategies in Chapters 8, 9, and 10 for recognizing his errors in logic and for dealing with the mental meltdowns he had been having off and on since he was a kid. He had given Chapter 4 only a little attention when he read through it the first time, but after working through the other chapters he went back to Chapter 4 to learn more about how to recognize his symptoms when they were mild and just beginning to return. Although he knew himself pretty well, he did not always recognize symptoms until they were severe and easily noticeable to others.

Paul found the idea that he could help manage his symptoms and even prevent recurrences by changing his reactions very appealing. It felt like a personal challenge, and he was determined to do whatever he could to keep his mood stable. Examples of how Paul worked through each exercise are provided throughout the workbook.

Raquel is 45 years old and has found a medication regimen that works well for her. She rarely has severe symptoms, and when they do occur she makes adjustments in her medication and in her actions to control them. She does a very good job of holding off the emergence of mania, but she still can become overwhelmed by stress, which usually leads to depression. She has struggled with low self-esteem much of her life, and when things go wrong she has a tendency to blame herself, feel hopeless, and cope by overeating, retreating to her bed, or refusing to interact with others. She wanted to learn how to control what she thought were overreactions to stress. What appealed most to Raquel were the sections in the workbook that focused more on the symptoms of depression. Like Amanda, she had a problem with negative thinking not only when she was depressed, but also when her stress level was high. Raquel put more effort into the exercises in Chapters 5, 8, and 9 than into the others. She was amazed to find out in Chapter 5 how many things she had been doing that probably worsened her depression. She also learned how to add positive experiences to her life and how to climb out of the rut of lethargy and procrastination.

Raquel was also very interested in learning to recognize when her emotions colored her thinking and how to avoid it or at least work through it. She always had a sense that her attitude could become very dark when she was depressed, but before reading Chapter 8 she thought she was the only person who experienced that. She recognized the thinking errors she made most often and learned the methods presented in Chapters 8 and 9 for straightening them out. Her responses to the exercises are provided throughout to give you an idea of how Raquel learned to control her reactions to stress.

Can You Do This on Your Own?

Learning the methods presented in this workbook is only part of what you need to manage your illness. Another important goal is finding a doctor you trust to help you determine the right medication regimen for you. Your doctor needs to be someone that you can be honest with about your symptoms and your adherence to medication treatment and from whom you can take candid feedback.

The majority of effort to manage your illness has to come from you. You can receive advice, instructions, and medications from others, but you're the one who has to do the work. You have to live with yourself from day to day, watch for signs that symptoms are returning, and take action to prevent it from happening. Others can support you, encourage you, and assist you if you're willing to let them, but **you have to take charge.**

➡ *What's Next?*

Now that you have an idea of how you can learn to gain control over your illness, it's time to get to work. In the next chapter you will begin to learn to recognize symptoms by gaining knowledge about the specific characteristics of depression and mania that have led to your diagnosis of bipolar disorder. If you're pretty familiar with how depression and mania are diagnosed, you might want to skip ahead to Chapter 3 and begin to chart your personal history.

Step 1

See It Coming

chapter two

Facts about Bipolar Disorder

In this chapter you will:

✓ Find out how a diagnosis of bipolar disorder is made.
✓ Learn about symptoms of major depression.
✓ Read a definition of mania and mixed episodes.
✓ See how street drugs, medications, and illnesses cause similar symptoms.

This chapter offers some basic information about bipolar disorder, including its diagnosis and related disorders. Although the description of the disorder provided cannot replace a thorough evaluation by a trained clinician,* it will give you an idea of how doctors go about deciding whether you have this illness.

How Did I Get the Diagnosis of Bipolar Disorder?

Bipolar disorder falls into a broader diagnostic category called *mood disorders*, according to the *Diagnostic and Statistical Manual of Mental Disorders* (DSM-IV-TR) published by the American Psychiatric Association in 2000. The DSM-IV-TR guidelines for making diagnoses have changed many times as researchers and clinicians have refined their understanding of the nature of mental illnesses. Each revision rep-

*Throughout the book I refer to your "doctor" or "therapist." For any given individual with bipolar disorder, however, the clinicians or practitioners who make psychiatric diagnoses, prescribe medication, and provide psychotherapy may be psychologists, psychiatrists, social workers, nurses, licensed professional counselors, marriage and family therapists, chemical dependency counselors, family practice/primary care doctors, interns in psychology, interns in social work, interns in counseling, medical residents, intake workers, and/or case workers.

So as to keep the text simple and straightforward—despite the fact that there are numerous types of professionals who provide care for individuals with bipolar disorder—I use the term "doctor" to describe anyone who prescribes medication and the term "therapist" for anyone who provides psychotherapy in any of its many forms. It is understood that the same individual might provide you with medication treatment and psychotherapy.

resents an improvement because it incorporates new scientific information about each disorder gathered since the writing of the last version. The DSM diagnosis guidelines include a list of symptoms that characterize the disorder and some guidelines for how long those symptoms must exist before a diagnosis can be made.

For all psychiatric disorders the specific symptoms have to occur together in time. For example, if your symptoms of mania included rapid speech, hyperactivity, and a euphoric mood, these symptoms would have to occur at the same time and last for a while to be considered clinically important. This rule is intended to keep clinicians from overdiagnosing things that everyone experiences from time to time. For example, some people talk fast. Everyone in their family talks fast or everyone from their part of the country talks fast. So talking fast would not necessarily be a symptom. Hyperactivity is also a matter of opinion. If you are easygoing and accustomed to low levels of noise and activity, someone who is highly energetic and raring to go might strike you as hyperactive instead of as just more hyper than you. And people can feel euphoric for short periods of time when good things are happening to them without being manic. **However, if symptoms of bipolar disorder:**

- occur together in time,
- differ from your normal self,
- cannot be explained away by a specific event or circumstance,
- persist for several days to several weeks, **and**
- have started to cause you some problems,

they are probably clinically significant, which means they may indicate that you have a psychiatric problem that needs attention.

Making a correct diagnosis of bipolar disorder is like putting together a puzzle. Information is collected and reviewed. After the pieces of the puzzle are assembled, the clinician looks for patterns. For example, your experiences might be compared to those of other people who have mood disorders to see if there are any similarities. To begin to gather clues a clinician would likely ask about changes in your mood, behavior, and thought processes. He or she would also be interested in your functioning at home and work, any new problems you've had, any illnesses that could have caused your symptoms, and your use of alcohol and street drugs. Clinicians will also want to know something about what you were like before the symptoms began. It is especially helpful at this point if family members or friends can give their observations about what you used to be like and how you have changed. If the clinician suspects that you have a medical problem unrelated to bipolar disorder that may be causing your symptoms, you might be asked to undergo some laboratory tests, such as a blood test. You can also expect questions about the psychiatric history of your family members. Mood disorders run in families. So if your mother had a mood disorder and an uncle had one, there is a chance that you have one too. Family history is another piece of the puzzle. Finally, an experienced clinician who is familiar with bipolar disorder will make observations about what he or she sees in your mood, your behavior, your speech pattern, and your thought processes. With this information in hand, the clinician will review the diagnostic guidelines for bipolar disorder in the DSM-IV-TR to see if you meet the criteria.

What Is Mania?

To be diagnosed with bipolar disorder, the DSM says you must have had **at least one manic episode** where alcohol, drugs of abuse, medications, or a general medical disorder did not cause the symptoms. For each symptom listed in the table on the following page, mark whether or not you have that symptom now or have had it in the past. If you're not sure, read about the symptom in the pages that follow and return to the table to mark your answer. At the end of the table you can determine whether you are currently manic or have been manic in the past.

The individual symptoms that make up the DSM-IV-TR criteria for a **manic episode** are presented in boxes on the following pages. An explanation of each symptom is provided following each box.

> *A distinct period of abnormally and persistently elevated, expansive, or irritable mood, lasting at least 1 week or requiring hospitalization.*

This is more than just a really good mood. This means feeling on top of the world, as if you couldn't possibly feel better, or feeling high like on drugs without having taken any. Or your mood can be so irritable that you're arguing with people, getting into fights, or can't stand the feel of your own skin. This euphoria or irritability is different from your normal mood, and it lasts all day for several days rather than being just a reaction to events in your life.

> *Three or more of the following symptoms are present (four with irritable vs. elevated or expansive mood).*

You have to have several symptoms at the same time so the clinician can be certain that this is really a clinically significant problem. Each individual item on the list is something that many people experience even if they do not have bipolar disorder. If only one or two symptoms were present, they would not be considered a problem and probably would not interfere with your everyday functioning.

The reason that four symptoms are required if you have an irritable rather than an expansive or elevated mood is that people get irritable, have trouble sleeping, and

Criteria for Diagnosis of Mania

Symptoms of mania	Had it in the past	Have it now	Not sure what it is
1. A distinct period of abnormally and persistently elevated, expansive, or irritable mood, lasting at least 1 week or requiring hospitalization.			Go to page 25.
2. Inflated self-esteem or grandiosity.			Go to page 27.
3. Decreased need for sleep.			Go to page 27.
4. More talkative than usual or pressure to keep talking.			Go to page 27.
5. Flight of ideas or subjective experience that thoughts are racing.			Go to page 28.
6. Distractibility.			Go to page 28.
7. An increase in goal-directed activity (either socially, at work or school, or sexually) or psychomotor agitation.			Go to page 28.
8. Excessive involvement in pleasurable activities that have a high potential for painful consequences.			Go to page 29.
Had or have five of these symptoms at the same time, and one of the symptoms is item 1 (only four if item 1 is elevated or expansive mood vs. irritable) AND			
It is not a mixed episode AND			Go to page 29.
The symptoms cause impaired functioning or need for hospitalization AND			Go to page 30.
The symptoms are not due to a general medical condition, substance abuse, or medications.			Go to page 30.
At least five symptoms were present and all the other conditions were met.	Past manic episode	Current manic episode	

Adapted with permission from the *Diagnostic and Statistical Manual of Mental Disorders* (4th ed., text rev.). Copyright 2000 American Psychiatric Association.

have poor concentration when they are depressed too. Requiring four symptoms helps clinicians be more certain that what is happening is actually a manic episode.

> *Inflated self-esteem or grandiosity.*

Inflated self-esteem is not just feeling better about yourself because you are not depressed anymore. The inflation goes beyond what would be considered normal. You might find yourself thinking that you're better, smarter, more creative, and more attractive than anyone you know. Or you might think that your ideas are the most brilliant ever, that they have no flaws, and that you're destined to get rich as a result. These claims could of course be true, but if there is no evidence to back up your claim and no one else agrees with you, or you normally have much lower self-esteem, feeling this way might be considered a symptom. Grandiosity is overconfidence taken to such a high level that you cannot see what is real and what is not.

> *Decreased need for sleep.*

If you have this symptom, you will find yourself feeling rested even though you are sleeping less than usual at night. You may have some trouble getting to sleep, but when you finally do, you sleep fewer hours than is normal for you. Or you might find yourself waking up much earlier than usual and being wide awake and unable to go back to sleep. If you usually get 7 to 8 hours of sleep, that amount might be reduced to 4 or 5 hours. Some people find they can't fall asleep at all when manic. What makes it a symptom of mania is that you seem to have enough energy to make it through the day even though you are sleeping less. In this sense it's different from the insomnia people experience when stressed or depressed. In those cases less sleep leaves people feeling exhausted. In mania, sometimes people do not feel the need to sleep until they have gone several days without it.

> *More talkative than usual or pressure to keep talking.*

This symptom tends to be more noticeable to others than to the person who has it. You may not feel like you're talking fast. In fact, it may seem to you that others are talking more slowly than usual. What you might notice is that you are tripping over your words or feeling tongue-tied because you're going too fast. You might even feel pressured to keep talking. What may be more noticeable are the comments from others that you're talking too much, jumping from subject to subject, or interrupting others when they are trying to take their turn to talk.

> *Flight of ideas or subjective experience that thoughts are racing.*

When racing thoughts are mild, it may seem like you just have more ideas or more thoughts running through your mind. The thoughts might seem at first to be more insightful or creative or to give you a sense that you really understand things that had previously eluded you. As this symptom progresses, you may find it hard to concentrate. Many people with bipolar disorder complain that they lose the ability to hold their thoughts together. They lose their train of thought too quickly and feel frustrated by this. They can also have trouble getting their ideas across to others. At their most extreme, racing thoughts can seem like they are going too fast to be expressed aloud. They stop making sense to you and no longer seem creative or brilliant. They bombard your mind, making it hard to have a conversation or even to fall asleep at night. You might want to turn them off, like turning off a radio, but you can't easily make them stop.

> *Distractibility.*

Distractibility is an annoying symptom that interferes with concentration, decision making, organization, and task completion. When this symptom occurs, you may find yourself distracted by external stimuli, like noise, lights, people, or activities going on around you. You might also be distracted by internal thoughts such as ideas, memories, urges to engage in new activities, or regrets. Others may notice that you seem to start projects or activities but get distracted and move on to something else before accomplishing the first. You may be moving around a lot, but not actually getting much completed because internal and external stimuli take your focus off what you are doing and direct your attention to something new.

> *An increase in goal-directed activity (either socially, at work or school, or sexually) or psychomotor agitation.*

Fueled by an increased number of ideas and greater energy than usual, many people find they are busier and more physically active when manic. If you've previously gone through an episode of depression during which you got behind on chores or other responsibilities, the extra energy and motivation that come at the beginning of mania can be highly welcomed. You feel the urge to do more and have the energy to do it. Problems come when racing thoughts and distractibility keep you from completing the tasks you've started or when impaired judgment leads you to take action in ways that could cause you problems down the line or be more than you can handle. Sometimes the activity starts with a desire for change, like changing your hairstyle, the way your furniture is arranged, or your job. If the change is big and is made impulsively, like quitting a job to start another career, it may create new problems and stress.

Psychomotor agitation is a term used to describe another form of increased activity. It is not directed toward a goal. It is like an excess of nervous energy. You may have difficulty sitting still or feel uncomfortable and irritated if you have to force yourself to do so. This restless feeling can appear at first as small repetitive movements like tapping your foot or biting your nails, but it usually progresses to pacing, rocking, or other kinds of action that help burn off some of this excessive nervous energy.

> *Excessive involvement in pleasurable activities that have a high potential for painful consequences.*

This is the symptom that usually catches the attention of family, friends, police officers, and health care providers. It includes spending sprees in which you might spend more than you can afford, buy items you do not need, or find yourself buying several of the same items for no particularly good reason. Driving too fast and taking more risks on the road than is normal for you is another form this symptom may take. It can and often does result in speeding tickets, arrests, or accidents. Drinking excessively and using illegal drugs also would fall into this symptom category, as would being more sexually active than usual. It is not unusual during a manic episode to engage in sexual activities that would be considered out of character for you.

> *It is not a mixed episode.*

A mixed episode is one in which you either alternate between depression and mania within hours or a few days or have symptoms of depression and mania simultaneously. This usually looks like hyperactivity and agitation with negative thoughts and irritability. It is an extremely uncomfortable state without the momentary joys that can come with a euphoric mania. A mixed episode is not a manic episode, but because the symptoms overlap, it can easily be mistaken for one. For example, if you were having the type of mixed episode in which you fluctuated rapidly between depression and mania, and a clinician saw you for the few hours you were feeling manic and not depressed, you could mistakenly be diagnosed with mania.

This criterion was included to remind clinicians to be thorough in their evaluation and to be alert to the possibility that a mixed state may be present.

> *The symptoms cause impaired functioning or need for hospitalization.*

Hypomania is a less severe state of mania (*hypo-* means "less than" or "under"). Hypomanic episodes cause most of the symptoms already described. However, when in this state, most people are still fully aware of the changes they are going through, and they don't act on the urges or impulses that are going through their minds. What best distinguishes mania from hypomania is the amount of impairment it causes. Mania is usually diagnosed when the symptoms are present and are severe enough to cause significant problems or are severe enough that you might need to be hospitalized to stay safe. These problems can include going into significant debt due to spending sprees, sexual promiscuity that caused relationship problems or health problems, reckless driving that caused accidents, impulsively quitting a job without a plan to support yourself, or even running away from home and neglecting your responsibilities. In contrast, during a hypomanic episode, you may have the symptoms listed for mania and also the desire to run away, spend money, or have an affair, but you stay in control and don't take those actions.

If manic symptoms are severe enough to require hospitalization, it's usually because you're too sick to take medications on your own, you're suicidal, you're too impaired to take care of your own basic needs, you can't fall asleep and as a result are becoming physically ill, you have forgotten to eat and are malnourished, or you are highly irritable and are making threats to harm others. Usually, if you have had mania before, you might become aware that you can't manage at home alone, you need medication to induce sleep, you're not clear-minded enough to handle your medications, or you might fear doing something stupid or dangerous and causing harm to yourself or to others. In those cases you might request hospitalization yourself. However, more often it is family or friends who recognize the severity of the symptoms and call for help.

> *The symptoms are not due to a general medical condition, substance abuse, or medications.*

If you had the symptoms of mania, but they were caused by a medical problem, a medication, or substances of abuse, you would be diagnosed with what is called a *mood disorder due to a general medical condition* or a *mood disorder due to substance abuse*. This would not be considered a true manic episode. If this was the only time you were manic, you would not qualify for a diagnosis of bipolar disorder. However, it is not uncommon for a person to have had a true manic episode at one time in life and a manic episode that was due to a general medical condition at another time in life. When this is the case, the diagnosis stands at bipolar disorder, but the treatment would involve resolution of the general medical condition and not just treatment of the symptoms of mania.

- *Medical conditions* that can cause manic-like symptoms include degenerative neurological diseases such as Huntington's disease or multiple sclerosis, strokes, vitamin deficiencies, hyperthyroidism, infections, and some cancers.
- *Substances of abuse* that can cause manic-like symptoms include alcohol, amphetamines, cocaine, hallucinogens, inhalants, opioids, sedatives, hypnotics, and anxiolytics.
- *Medications* that can cause manic-like symptoms include antidepressant medications of all types, corticosteroids, anabolic steroids, antiparkinson medications, and some decongestants.

What Is Major Depression?

Most people who have bipolar disorder have suffered through episodes of depression as well as mania. There are many forms and subtypes of depression, but the one that people with bipolar disorder have is called *major depression*. The word *major* isn't intended to imply that the depression is terrible or the worst possible type; it is used simply to distinguish this diagnosable depression from the minor depressions that everyone has. Clinicians usually refer to major depression in people who have bipolar disorder as *bipolar depression*; they call it *unipolar depression* in people who have never had mania or hypomania. *Unipolar* means "one end." This means you feel the lows of major depression but never have the highs of mania. *Bipolar* means "two ends"—up and down. This means you have experienced the highs of mania at some point in your life as well as the lows of major depression.

The DSM-IV-TR criteria for major depression are listed in the table on the next page. Place a check next to each symptom you currently have or have had in the past. If you're not sure, read about the symptom in the sections that follow.

The individual symptoms that make up the DSM-IV-TR criteria for an **episode of depression** are presented in boxes on the pages 33–38. An explanation of each symptom is provided following each box.

> *Five* or more of the following symptoms have been **present during the same two-week period** and represent a change from previous functioning. One of the five symptoms must be either depressed mood or loss of interest and pleasure.

There are several elements to this general rule worth noting.

- First, five symptoms must be present at the same time. That is because each individual symptom of major depression is something that many people experience from time to time when they are not depressed. To be certain that the symptoms are indicative of major depression, lots of them have to be present together.
- Second, the symptoms must last for at least 2 weeks before they are consid-

Criteria for Diagnosis of Major Depression

Symptoms of major depression	Had it in the past	Have it now	Not sure what it is
1. Depressed mood most of the day, nearly every day.			Go to page 33.
2. Markedly diminished interest or pleasure in all or almost all activities most of the day nearly every day.			Go to page 33.
3. Significant weight loss when not dieting, weight gain, loss of appetite, or increase in appetite that persists nearly every day.			Go to page 34.
4. Insomnia or hypersomnia nearly every day.			Go to page 34.
5. Psychomotor agitation or retardation nearly every day.			Go to page 35.
6. Fatigue or loss of energy nearly every day.			Go to page 35.
7. Feelings of worthlessness or excessive or inappropriate guilt.			Go to page 36.
8. Diminished ability to think or concentrate or indecisiveness nearly every day.			Go to page 36.
9. Recurrent thoughts of death, suicidal ideation without a specific plan, a suicide attempt, or a specific plan for committing suicide.			Go to page 37.
Had or have five of these symptoms at the same time and one of the symptoms is item 1 or 2 **AND**			
The symptoms cause impaired functioning or need for hospitalization **AND**			Go to page 37.
The symptoms are not due to a general medical condition, substance abuse, or medications **AND**			Go to page 38.
It is not bereavement.			
At least five symptoms were present and all the other conditions were met.	Past major depressive episode	Current major depressive episode	

Adapted with permission from the *Diagnostic and Statistical Manual of Mental Disorders* (4th ed., text rev.). Copyright 2000 American Psychiatric Association.

ered clinically important. This keeps clinicians from making the mistake of diagnosing depression when it may be only a normal reaction to stress, moodiness caused by hormone fluctuations, or symptoms caused by a brief medical illness.

• Third, the symptoms have to be different from the person's usual self. This is a tricky one because some people have been depressed for so long that it has become normal for them or they've forgotten what normal feels like. It is clearly not normal to have five or more symptoms of depression at the same time. To sort it out, more clues might be needed, such as family history of depression or bipolar disorder.

• Fourth, one of the five symptoms has to be depressed mood or loss of interest. This rule was included because major depression is experienced primarily as a change in emotion and desire. If you are happy and have the other physical symptoms of major depression, chances are you have something else wrong with you such as a thyroid problem, poorly controlled diabetes, or a virus.

> *Depressed mood most of the day, nearly every day.*

The quality of depressed mood can vary greatly from person to person. Some people feel sad and are tearful, like they might feel if they were grieving. Others feel an emptiness, loneliness, or darkness like no other sadness they have ever felt. Some people feel a lack of emotion or feel neutral. It's not unusual for depressed mood to be mixed with irritability, anger, or anxiety, particularly for men and for children and adolescents. For the most severe forms of major depression that don't improve easily with medication, the sad mood will not lift even if something good is happening. Those who experience this level of sadness say they know intellectually when something good is happening, but they don't feel any joy or happiness inside. Others have the ability to respond momentarily when good things happen. This is called a *reactive mood*. They perk up while the event is occurring, such as during a celebration, when hearing good news, or when a loved one visits. But when the event is over, their mood quickly returns to sadness.

> *Markedly diminished interest or pleasure in all or almost all activities most of the day nearly every day.*

When inquiring about this symptom, most depressed people say they have not had the energy to do anything pleasurable or interesting in some time. That makes it hard for them to know if they have lost interest or are just too tired or unmotivated to take part in activities. Loss of interest or pleasure is not limited to big events like vacations or parties. It's usually noticeable during everyday events and includes enjoying work less than usual and not wanting to play with the kids, visit with friends, or spend time on hobbies. When pleasure and interest have diminished, most people notice that they've been avoiding phone calls from friends, do not read books as much as usual, don't really want to hear about other people's activities, and take little or no pleasure in eating, watching television, or going to movies. It's important to distinguish loss of interest and pleasure from loss of energy. When it is a motivation and interest problem, there is no desire to participate in activities, even when you have the energy to do so.

> *Significant weight loss when not dieting, weight gain, loss of appetite, or increase in appetite that persists nearly every day.*

Logically it seems that a decrease in appetite should lead to weight loss and an increase in appetite should lead to weight gain, but for a variety of reasons this is not always the case. You can have no appetite but might eat anyway. In fact, when people are feeling down, they will often eat comfort foods, which are foods that usually make them feel better. Sweets, soft foods that take little effort to eat, or foods from your childhood are examples of comfort foods. Another form this symptom can take is less enjoyment of food than usual or loss of taste for certain things, even though the amount eaten may not change. Some people have a surge in their appetite when depressed and find themselves eating even when not hungry.

Overeating can obviously cause an increase in weight, but decreases in activity from loss of interest or low energy can reduce calorie burn and also lead to weight gain even when calorie intake stays about the same. For children or adolescents weight might not change at all; but this can still be considered a symptom because as they grow they are expected to increase proportionally in weight.

> *Insomnia or hypersomnia nearly every day.*

There are three basic types of insomnia. One type is called *initial insomnia*. This occurs when you have more trouble falling asleep than is normal for you. Less than 30 minutes is generally considered a normal amount of time to fall asleep, assuming that you're going to bed at your usual time. Initial insomnia is so frustrating that some people deal with it by not going to bed until they are extremely exhausted or by engaging in some other activity like reading or watching television or surfing the Internet until they feel tired enough to fall asleep. When they finally turn out the lights to sleep, they may fall asleep quickly, but much later than they usually would choose to fall asleep.

Middle insomnia, the second type, occurs when you wake up during the night and may have trouble getting back to sleep. When middle insomnia is severe, people wake up several times each night. When they do sleep, their sleep is fitful and not restful. They awake feeling tired. Waking up to use the bathroom, get a drink of water, or check on a noise that woke you is not considered insomnia if you can go back to sleep quickly.

The third type of insomnia is called *terminal insomnia* or *early morning awakening*. This occurs when you wake up an hour or more earlier in the morning than intended and cannot go back to sleep. Many people have an internal system and wake themselves up without an alarm clock or just before the alarm is ready to ring. It is considered terminal insomnia only if the time they wake up is much earlier than usual.

Hypersomnia is the opposite problem, sleeping much more than normal. Hypersomnia can include going to bed a lot earlier than usual, taking naps during the day, or feeling sleepy throughout the day despite getting enough sleep. With hypersomnia, sleep is usually fairly sound but causes problems because you're sleeping rather than engaging in other activities such as interacting with others, doing chores, or having fun.

Psychomotor agitation or retardation nearly every day.

Psychomotor agitation includes restlessness, pacing, and generally having difficulty sitting still for long periods of time. You might find yourself getting up and walking around at work more often than usual, having trouble sitting through a movie, or preferring movement to inactivity despite being tired. If you don't give in to the urge to move around, you may feel irritable, lose your focus or concentration, or find that you can't stand the feel of your own skin.

Psychomotor retardation can include slowness in movement, thought, or speech. Some people report feeling like they are in slow motion. It takes longer for them to complete tasks. They literally walk more slowly than usual and find themselves sitting still for long periods of time. Slowness in speech can include having difficulty finding the right words to say, speaking slowly, or taking a longer time than usual to respond to questions. It feels like the mental wheels in your brain are moving slowly. If you usually move and talk fast, it may be harder to detect psychomotor retardation, especially if slowing down makes you more like the average person. You will probably notice that you are not as sharp, quick-minded, or quick-witted as usual, but others may not notice the difference.

Fatigue or loss of energy nearly every day.

Loss of energy is one of the first things that people notice when they are getting depressed. They tire more easily than usual, running out of steam to complete normal activities. Even after getting enough sleep, depression can make you feel tired, but if coupled with insomnia, the low energy is worse. As mentioned earlier, in the section on loss of interest and pleasure, it is easy to confuse lack of motivation and lack of energy. You can have the desire but lack the physical energy to engage in your normal routine. People who have this symptom say that they want to clean their house, wash their car, or buy groceries, but they don't have enough energy to do it on their own.

Feelings of worthlessness or excessive or inappropriate guilt.

Some people are always hard on themselves. They report having low self-esteem, feel like they've fallen short of their potential, or have excessively high standards that they have trouble meeting. This is not the same thing as feelings of worthlessness. Worthlessness is when you feel you have less value as a human being than others. You think you're just taking up space and your existence is meaningless. This is much worse than what we would normally consider low self-esteem or self-criticism. People with this symptom say that they are nothing, unworthy, and unlovable, and encouragement from others does not change their minds.

Excessive guilt is when you blame yourself for significant things that are not entirely your fault, failing to see the complexity of the situation or the shared responsibility of others. Excessive guilt can also include holding on to regrets for events that occurred long ago that cannot be changed, resolved, or set right. This should not be confused with having a normal conscience and regretting choices made in life. Those with excessive guilt blame themselves for things they had no control over, or they find errors or faults so unacceptable that they ruminate about them on a regular basis for months or even years at a time. They seem to accumulate a mental list of errors and wrongdoings that can never be forgiven or forgotten. They are usually able to forgive the sins of others and excuse their faults, but hold a double standard and cannot relieve themselves of guilt.

Diminished ability to think or concentrate or indecisiveness nearly every day.

Those who suffer from poor concentration and indecisiveness find it difficult to read or follow the story line of a movie or television show. They have to reread paragraphs of a newspaper or magazine story because they lose their train of thought. Sometimes this is because their mind wanders to related issues, ideas, people, or events or their mind gets flooded with negative thoughts and worries.

One way decision making can become impaired is that you can't organize your thoughts well enough to define the problem clearly or to consider all your options. Another reason is that self-doubt creeps in and you become afraid that you'll make a bad decision. You reason to yourself that making no decision is better than making a bad decision and suffering the consequences. Sometimes decision making is a problem because the negative and hopeless thinking that accompanies depression makes every alternative seem unreasonable or untenable. Many times there are multiple problems that you are facing at the same time and you are looking for a solution that can resolve several issues at a time and make the pieces of your life fall into place. This is more a fantasy than a reality because it is rare that you can solve all your problems with one intervention. Looking for the "right answer" or the "best choice" may keep you from choosing and implementing a solution. If you find that this is becoming a pattern with you, then you probably have this symptom.

It is not only the big decisions that can be hard to make when you're depressed. Smaller decisions about what to wear, what to eat, or what to do first can also seem more complicated, difficult, or burdensome than usual. You might find yourself staring into the refrigerator for long periods of time, ultimately choosing nothing because you can't make up your mind. You might stand in front of your open closet and not know what to wear even after trying on several different things. You might find yourself flipping through the television channels several times and finding nothing you want to watch. It can feel like there are too many choices and too many decisions to make and you would be happier if someone would just make a few for you.

> *Recurrent thoughts of death, suicidal ideation without a specific plan, a suicide attempt, or a specific plan for committing suicide.*

When depression is severe and nothing seems to make it better, people think about death as an alternative. They are in emotional pain and believe that one way to relieve the pain is to no longer exist. This is a dangerous fantasy that many people share. Sometimes these thoughts are very specific, involving a specific plan to kill themselves and ideas for when to do so. More often, however, suicidal thoughts are more vague or general. No plan has been made, and the person is pretty certain that he or she will not do it, but thinking about the possibility brings some peace, as if it means there is a way out of the discomfort. Other forms this symptom takes include desires to disappear, to fall asleep and never wake up, or to contract an incurable illness that takes them quickly. A milder form involves not caring if you live or die or believing that life is not worth living.

> *The symptoms cause impaired functioning or need for hospitalization.*

The symptoms of depression must be bothersome or interfere with your usual level of functioning to be considered clinically significant. This criterion is sometimes difficult to meet in people whose usual level of functioning is quite high. Impairment brings them down to a lower level but still leaves them in good enough shape to make it through each day. In this case, the criterion is satisfied when people are greatly troubled by the symptoms or the extra effort to cope is beginning to wear them out or they find themselves losing their ability to "fake it."

The symptoms are not due to a general medical condition, substance abuse, or medications.

As with any other psychiatric illness, it's important not to confuse major depression with symptoms caused by some other biological process such as a general medical condition or illness, treatment for it, or a side effect of substance abuse.

- *Medical conditions* that can be mistaken for depression include neurological illnesses such as Parkinson's disease, stroke, vitamin deficiencies, endocrine problems such as hypothyroidism, infections, hepatitis, mononucleosis, or cancer.
- *Substances of abuse* that can cause symptoms of depression include alcohol, amphetamines, cocaine, hallucinogens, opioids, sedatives, or inhalants.
- *Medications* such as antihypertensives, oral contraceptives, anabolic steroids, anticancer agents, analgesics, and cardiac medications can also produce depression-like symptoms.

It is not bereavement.

Bereavement is another word for grief after a loss. It is normal to have some of the symptoms of depression after suffering a great loss. The most common loss is the death of a loved one, but losses can also include divorce, moving away from home, losing a job, or losing a pet. Sadness, tearfulness, anxiety, sleep problems, and loss of energy or appetite are the most common symptoms. Usually these symptoms begin to resolve within a few weeks and have subsided to a great degree within two months of the loss. Grief, however, can turn into a major depressive episode if it lingers longer than two months or if the symptoms become more severe and interfere with your ability to manage your responsibilities. Those who have had major depression in the past are at a higher risk for becoming clinically depressed after suffering a loss. The way clinicians tell the difference between bereavement (sometimes called *uncomplicated bereavement*) and major depression has to do with the type and severity of symptoms experienced. When a person begins to have suicidal thoughts, feels worthless, slows down physically and mentally, begins to hear voices or see visions, and cannot function normally at home or at work, it is no longer considered bereavement. It is classified as major depression.

⇒ *What's Next?*

The diagnostic criteria presented in this chapter give you an idea of how clinicians diagnose bipolar disorder. In addition to the symptoms that make up the guidelines for diagnosis, there are many other more subtle symptoms of depression and mania. As you learn more about the signs that your symptoms may be returning, you will have a better chance of stopping them before they worsen. The next step is to use the information from this chapter to help you construct a life chart of your history of bipolar disorder. Once you have the big picture, you may be able to identify patterns that will help you predict when the next episode of depression or mania may occur. If you can see it coming and act quickly, you have a good chance of preventing symptoms from getting out of control.

chapter three

Charting Your Personal History

In this chapter you will:

✓ Create your own life chart.
✓ Learn to identify important patterns in your life course with bipolar disorder.
✓ Make predictions about future episodes of depression and mania.
✓ Begin to keep a diary of your treatment history.

Whether you have only recently been diagnosed or have struggled with this illness for a while, it's only natural to try to make sense of the events of your life, the ups and downs, the turning points, and the problems. If you've had bipolar disorder for some time, the episodes of depression and mania can seem to run together after a while and get so mixed with life events, treatments, and other efforts to alter your mood that it can be difficult to determine what's what. For example, did you get depressed because you were drinking, or were you drinking because you were feeling depressed and couldn't sleep? Did the stress of a relationship ending throw you into a manic state, or did a manic state make you act in ways that caused the relationship to end? Did the medication flip you into mania when you had been feeling depressed, or was that just the natural course of the illness? These questions are hard to answer yet important to consider.

When you know more about your personal history of bipolar disorder, you have the beginnings of a roadmap to help you prevent future episodes or control the course of your illness. If you've had a number of episodes, you can learn from those experiences what types of factors make you more vulnerable to becoming depressed or manic. With that information in hand, you can take precautions to avoid these triggers or at least be better prepared to handle them when they arise. If you know what the symptoms of depression or mania look like when mild, you can see them coming and stop them before they worsen. And if you have a good idea of how medication affects you, it will be easier for you to communicate your needs to your doctor when symptoms begin to emerge or to work out a preventive plan for the early stages of recurrence of depression or mania. The more you know about yourself, the better equipped you will be to take control of your illness.

Life Charting

One method for trying to make sense of the events in your life related to bipolar disorder is to use a Life Chart. Life-charting methods were developed by Dr. Robert Post at the National Institute of Mental Health and have been an important tool in research on the effects of starting and stopping medication for bipolar disorder. Life Charts are also used to help professionals make accurate diagnoses. They put on a time line the sequence of events in your life that relate to bipolar disorder, such as time of illness and wellness, treatments, hospitalizations, major life events, medical conditions, and periods of excessive alcohol use or substance abuse. The sequence of events helps doctors and therapists sort out causes and effects of depression and mania, identify triggers of relapse, and understand which treatments have been effective or ineffective in controlling symptoms and preventing relapse.

The main value of knowing your common patterns is that you are in a better place to predict when the next episode is likely to occur so you can take precautions to keep it from happening. This might be difficult if you have had only a few episodes and have not had enough experience with the illness to identify patterns. However, the newly diagnosed person with bipolar disorder is in the best position to begin constructing a Life Chart that can be kept over time. An up-to-date account of episodes of depression and mania will be more accurate than one pieced together through memory.

Another advantage of creating your Life Chart is that you can get a better handle on the big picture. If you're like many other people who have bipolar disorder, you may struggle with so many daily ups and downs that you find it hard to see discrete periods of depression and mania. When your life of ups and downs seems like a blur, you can get the sense that you have no control over it. Looking more closely at the patterns can give you ideas for how you might take control over this illness rather than feeling out of control.

Preparing to Create Your Life Chart

Before you begin to draw you own Life Chart, there are a few facts that might be helpful to know.

- Life charts of bipolar disorder show periods of depression, mania, hypomania, and mixed states. These periods of illness are called *episodes*.
- An episode is a single period of depression, mania, or hypomania from beginning to end. This means that you had no symptoms before the episode began and you felt OK after the symptoms went away.
- Episodes can last anywhere from several weeks to several months. In some cases, symptoms can persist for years if not treated properly.
- Most people who have bipolar disorder have several episodes of depression, mania, mixed states, and hypomania during their lifetime, sometimes with years of perfect wellness between episodes.
- Episodes can begin after a big stress or a change in your life. But they can also occur for no reason at all.

The life-charting process distinguishes not only between periods of depression and mania, but also between periods of feeling normal, without symptoms, and periods of feeling symptomatic. If you are like Raquel and have had long periods of time when you have had no symptoms, you may have a clear picture of what normal is like. However, if you are more like Paul, who seems to have lots of minor ups and downs between full episodes of depression and mania, you may have forgotten what you are like when normal. Or you might feel like Amanda, who sometimes thinks that feeling bad is normal for her. Before you begin creating your Life Chart, take a moment to think about what it feels like to be without symptoms and jot down your ideas on Worksheet 3.1.

The sample Life Chart at the bottom of the facing page belongs to 45-year-old Raquel, who is married and the mother of two children and has bipolar disorder.

Raquel experienced her first episode of depression at age 15 after her girlfriend died in a car accident. It lasted almost a year, but she was able to get back on her feet and finish high school. At age 19 she had her first manic episode, after the birth of her daughter. Her obstetrician thought her agitation and inability to sleep were probably due to her hormones readjusting and did not think she needed treatment. Unfortunately, after just a few weeks of manic symptoms she fell into a severe depression. She was frightened by thoughts of suicide that kept going through her mind, so she went to see her doctor and he put her on an antidepressant medication. The medication seemed to work, and her depression went away after about 6 months. Once she was back to normal, she stopped taking the antidepressants. Two years later, at age 21, Raquel had her third episode of depression. She and her boyfriend broke up after she found out he had been with someone else. She thought she would feel better once he moved out, but unfortunately, even after he left, her symptoms of depression continued. She went back to her doctor, and he put her back on the same antidepressant medicine she had taken before, but this time the result was different. Within only a few days of taking the medication she felt a lot better. It

| worksheet 3.1 | **What Normal Is Like for Me** |

What normal is like for me:

Mood:

Energy level:

Attitude:

Actions:

From *The Bipolar Workbook* by Monica Ramirez Basco. Copyright 2006 by The Guilford Press. Permission to photocopy this form is granted to purchasers of this book for personal use only (see copyright page for details).

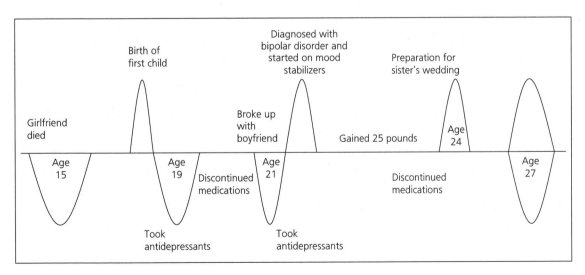

Raquel's Life Chart—Part 1.

seemed like a miracle at first, but as her mood continued to climb she became hyperactive, didn't feel the need to sleep, and wouldn't stop talking. Her mom called the doctor, and within a few days she was hospitalized for mania. After evaluating Raquel and hearing about her reaction to antidepressant medications, the psychiatrist diagnosed her condition as bipolar disorder. He prescribed medication to stabilize her mood and to help her sleep. She went home after 5 days in the hospital and continued to take the medication off and on for several years, but managed to stay out of the hospital and avoid severe relapses of depression and mania until she went off her medication many years later, after getting disgusted with her weight gain.

It began one day when Raquel went shopping for a new dress for her sister's wedding. She looked at herself in the mirror and at the 25 pounds she had gained while on the medication and decided to stop taking it. A few weeks later, she began to drop weight and felt better than she had in months. The good feeling increased so slowly that at first it was barely noticeable to her or to others. Feeling more energetic, she was able to do more with her daughter, keep her apartment clean, and helped out with wedding preparations. She bought a new computer and taught herself how to use a number of office work programs. Each night she waited until her daughter was off the computer so she could play games and write letters to her friends. She was glad to be able to establish contact with friends who had moved away since their college years. Since she had little time to herself during the day, she would work on her computer until the early-morning hours even though she had to get up early to tend to her daughter.

Raquel got less and less sleep as time when on. Sleep loss turned her perkiness into hyperactivity. She became very disorganized and talked so fast that her family couldn't understand her. When her mom confronted her with these symptoms, Raquel admitted that she was getting manic. With her doctor's help, Raquel was hospitalized once again. Although she recovered, she hated her hospital stay and vowed to herself and her family that she would stay on the medication to avoid ever having to go back. Several years later, she once again discontinued her lithium against the advice of her psychiatrist and the pattern repeated itself. This time her symptoms evolved into a mixed episode.

The Life Chart presents a representation of Raquel's story on a time line. It shows the sequence of events in a way that illustrates how her illness progressed, the things that made it better, such as medication and hospitalization, and the things that made it worse, such as childbirth, relationship stress, and discontinuing use of her mood-stabilizing medications. Seeing her Life Chart helped Raquel understand how her episodes began and ended and how medications can help. She made the decision to stay on medication for as long as necessary to avoid another manic episode. Her Life Chart following this time period is shown in the figure on the facing page.

Raquel got married and had a second child without developing postpartum depression or mania. She and her doctor had worked out a plan for discontinuing

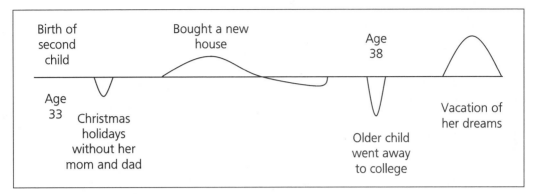

Raquel's Life Chart—Part 2.

medication prior to pregnancy and throughout her first trimester. Medications were resumed when her doctor felt that it would be safe for the baby. She had a short low period during the holidays because she missed her mom and dad, who had moved out of state the prior year. The excitement and stress of buying her first home accounted for her next set of mood changes, but she never got fully manic or depressed. When her older daughter left for college, she felt very depressed for several weeks, but with some additional psychotherapy she was able to get back on her feet in no time. Recently, Raquel went on the trip of a lifetime, a week in New York with her husband. She was elated during this time and for several weeks thereafter, but was not hypomanic. She had kept her commitment to staying on medication and learned to identify the return of symptoms. She worked with her doctor and her therapist as she needed and avoided a full relapse into depression and mania.

How to Create Your Own Life Chart

Use the Life Chart pages provided for you in Worksheet 3.2 or use scrap paper to make a first draft before drawing the final version in your workbook. Draw a line across the middle of the page. This is your time line. Points on this line represent feeling fine. Anything drawn below the line represents depression. Anything drawn above the line represents mania. The figure on page 47 provides some examples of how to draw episodes of depression and mania on your Life Chart.

• **Step 1: Draw in the episodes of depression and mania.** It is usually easiest to start at the present time and work backward on the time line. For example, if you are currently in an episode of depression that began last December, you would draw a depressive episode like the ones in the figure without the line going all the way back up to the normal level. Mark December on the chart where the episode starts and today's date for where you are now. If you have had major depressions or

Life Chart

The line represents the passage of time from the beginning of your illness to the present. Use the sample episodes from the figure on page 47 to draw your pattern of depression and mania over time.

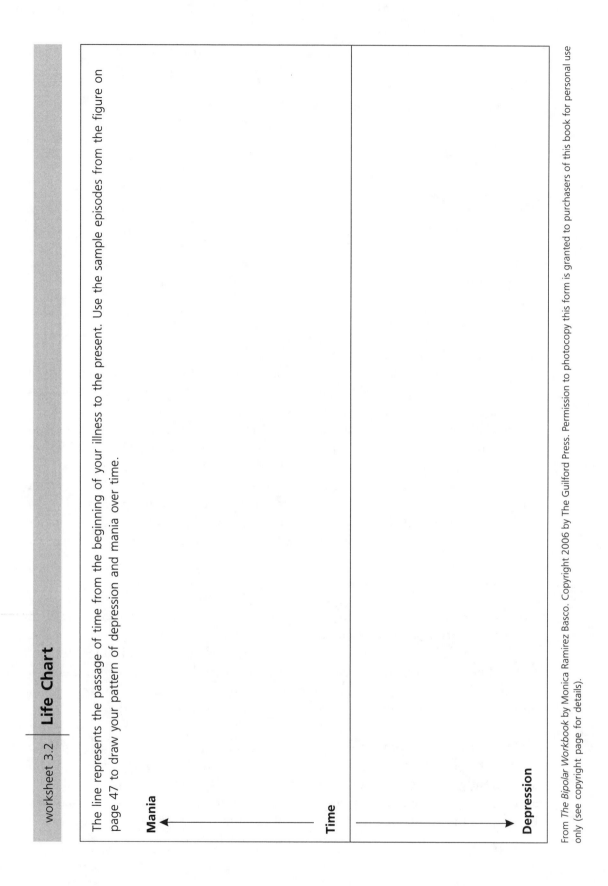

Mania

Time

Depression

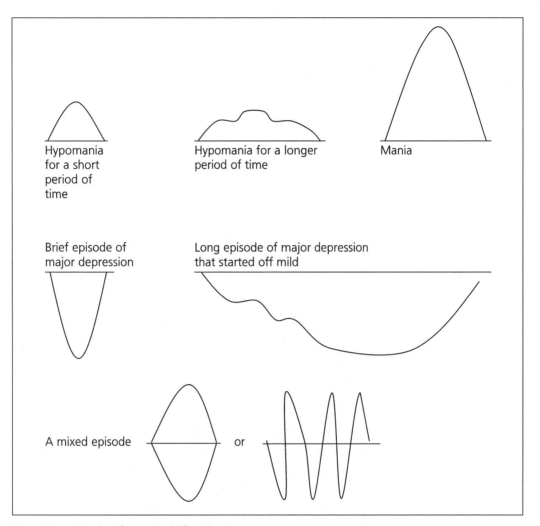

Sample episodes for your Life Chart.

manic episodes in the past, draw those on the line and write in the approximate dates when they occurred. If you can't remember the date, try to recall how old you would have been at the time. If you have had bipolar disorder for a long time, you may not be able to recall every time you've been ill. In that case, it's easiest to create a Life Chart for just the past few years.

• **Step 2: Add in periods of time when you used alcohol excessively or when you might have used street drugs.** You can fill this in on the time line any way you would like. It may be easiest to mark these time periods below the episodes of depression, mania, hypomania, or mixed episodes, as in the example in the next figure (page 48).

• **Step 3: Mark on the line when major life events occurred.** Major life events

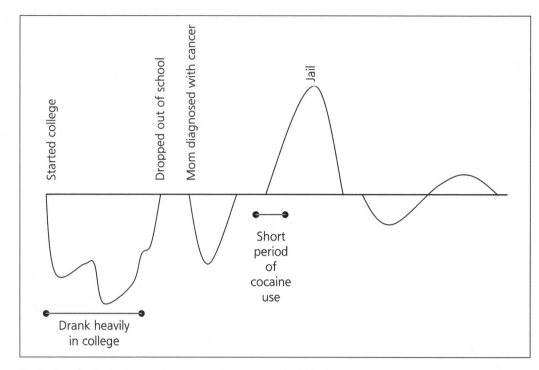

Periods of alcohol or substance abuse on the Life Chart.

include starting or stopping school, losses, job changes, marriage, birth of children, changing residences, and accidents. Be sure to include major medical problems such as diabetes or hypertension as well as injuries, surgeries, and any physical problem that you consider bothersome or important.

• **Step 4: Include information about times of treatment.** Each time a hospitalization occurred, mark the point on the Life Chart with an **H**. If you were treated in an emergency room, mark **ER** on the time line. Add in times when you took medication and when you stopped using medication. If you still remember, write in the name of the medication you were taking.

If you need help in completing your Life Chart, take your first draft to your doctor and ask him or her to help you add in treatment information and dates of each episode. You may have a family member or friend who remembers the approximate dates and can help you fill in the details.

• **Step 5: Make a note on your Life Chart when other psychological problems may have occurred.** It's fairly common to have other psychiatric or psychological difficulties in addition to bipolar disorder. In fact, the majority of people with bipolar disorder have at least one other disorder. The most common ones are alcohol and substance abuse, but also occurring quite frequently are anxiety and eating disorders. Anxiety disorders that you might have experienced in your life include panic attacks, social phobia, obsessive–compulsive disorder, and simple phobias like fear of heights. Eating disorders can include anorexia, bulimia, or binge eating disorders. If you are uncertain whether you have had any conditions, ask your doctor or therapist.

What Does It All Mean?

Now that you've completed your Life Chart, it's time to analyze the picture. Following is a list of questions to ask yourself about the patterns you see.

• **Are there any obvious patterns of depressive episodes or manic episodes on your life chart?** Do they always seem to come on at the same time of the year? This is called a *seasonal pattern*. Episodes that start at about the same times of the year and end at about the same times of the year suggest that your illness is sensitive to seasonal changes. The most common seasonal pattern is to get depressed during the late fall and winter months when the days are short and the nights are long. In the spring, when the days are getting longer and the nights shorter, hypomania and mania often emerge. If you see a seasonal pattern, you can probably predict when the next episode will occur. Preparations can be made to prevent those symptoms from returning or at least for catching them early. Look over your Life Chart and mark your observations on Worksheet 3.3.

• **Is there an association between the occurrence of stressful events and the onset of depression or mania?** It's not unusual for the first few depressive, manic, hypomanic, or mixed episodes to follow a stressful or life-altering event. This includes external events like the death of a family member or internal events like an injury or medical illness. However, after the first few, it is less likely that episodes will be linked to stressful events. This does not mean that stressful events are no longer bothersome. It just means there are many other reasons for the return of symptoms. Finding your unique triggers for the return of depression or mania will be a goal of the remaining chapters of this book. Write down your initial impressions on Worksheets 3.4 and 3.5.

• **Is there a connection between treatments and episodes?** You might find on your Life Chart that medications were started after an episode began and they helped to control your symptoms. Treatments may have been initiated in the hospital or an emergency room or during a regularly scheduled visit with your doctor. Perhaps some medications were more effective than others. Knowing which medications work for you is very important, as is knowing which do not work and which caused especially unpleasant side effects. Worksheet 3.8, called Your Treatment History, is provided later in this chapter (page 57) for keeping track of your reactions to medications.

Another question to ask yourself about medications and your Life Chart is

| worksheet 3.3 | **Seasonal Patterns in Depression and Mania** |

What patterns do I see in my episodes of depression and mania?

Seasonal patterns?

Is it weather related?

Are there common events associated with symptoms?

Amanda's Worksheet 3.3

What patterns do I see in my episodes of depression and mania?

Seasonal patterns?

I always seem to get more depressed around Thanksgiving and manic around Easter. I never thought of it as seasonal, but maybe it is.

Is it weather related?

It usually starts to snow by Thanksgiving. I thought it was the pressure of the holidays and being stuck in the house that made me depressed.

Are there common events associated with symptoms?

The holidays.

worksheet 3.4	**Situations That Trigger Depression**

Situations that seem to trigger depression

Relationship events?

Losses?

Changes in my life?

Illness or childbirth?

Other things?

Raquel's Worksheet 3.4

Situations that seem to trigger depression

Relationship events?

Fights with my husband get me depressed.

Losses?

When my best friend died, I had my first serious depression.

Changes in my life?

Just the ones I already listed.

Illness or childbirth?

I have had depression and mania after giving birth. I'm not having any more kids, so this is not an issue.

Other things?

Rainy days.

---

worksheet 3.5 | **Situations That Trigger Mania**

Situations that seem to trigger mania

Vacations?

Schedule changes?

Moving to a new area?

Partying?

Other things?

Tommy's Worksheet 3.5

Situations that seem to trigger mania

Vacations?

No.

Schedule changes?

Not really.

Moving to a new area?

No.

Partying?

Maybe.

Other things?

Not sleeping for a couple of days.

whether you were taking medications regularly before each episode began. The most common cause of relapse in bipolar disorder is poor adherence to medication treatment. Poor adherence means not taking medication as it was prescribed, missing doses, decreasing the amounts, or stopping it altogether. While you may have very good reasons for altering your medication regimen on your own, doing so does put you at greater risk for relapse. Chapters 6 and 7 will help you get the most out of your medication and figure out how to cope with the unpleasant aspects of treatment. Make some notes on Worksheet 3.6 on any possible connections between taking or not taking medications and the return of symptoms.

Tommy, Paul, Amanda, and Raquel have all gone through times in their lives when they did not take prescribed medication. When Tommy was first diagnosed with bipolar disorder, he did not believe he had it. While he was in the hospital, he took medication as he was told, but as soon as he was back in his apartment on his own he stopped taking it. His parents would ask him about his medications because they could see that he was still not acting like his old self. Tommy would lie and say that he was taking it, and his parents would believe him. Within a few weeks Tommy would be manic again and would have to be hospitalized. Tommy was hos-

| worksheet 3.6 | **Treatment and Symptoms** |

Looking back on your Life Chart, do you see a connection between treatment and symptoms?

Do you function better when taking medication?

Do you do better when you are in therapy?

Are you not in treatment when symptoms start?

Do symptoms start when treatment is stopped?

Do antidepressants bring on mania?

---

pitalized four times within 7 months with each hospitalization increasing in length. His Life Chart would show that within a few weeks of stopping medication Tommy got manic. He is still young and has not gone off his medication since his last hospitalization. But there will be challenges ahead when he may take himself off medications again to see what will happen.

Paul started taking medication for bipolar disorder when he was just a kid. Acceptance of his diagnosis was never a question. His parents told him what he had and they gave him medicine for it. He took it regularly until he was in middle school. From eighth grade to his junior year, Paul and his parents were constantly debating about his medications. Paul no longer accepted their directions about lots of things, including taking medication. He rebelled and refused to take it for months at a time. What would bring him back to treatment was having a severe period of depression. It always took medication to get him out of it. In his junior year of high school he got drunk and tried to kill himself. He ran his car into a tree and suffered many injuries. Surgery, physical therapy, and medication brought him back to normal. Paul did not want to go to those depths of depression again, and he had learned that going off medication meant that depression would eventually return. His Life Chart would show that before his worst periods of depression he had discontinued his medication.

Amanda has had the most difficulty of the group sticking with medication. Although she does not always admit it, she "plays around" with her medication all the time. She experiments on her own with adding or reducing doses, adding natural supplements from time to time, and taking herself off some medications altogether. She has also had the most difficulty of the group controlling her symptoms of depression and mania. Especially since becoming a nurse and being educated about medicines, she has often thought that she knew more than her doctors about controlling her illness and would alter her regimen the way she thought was right. Sometimes she would make changes that seemed to help, and other times she made it worse.

Amanda really hates the idea of taking medication because it reminds her that she has bipolar disorder and is "not normal." Because she knows she is stuck with this illness forever, she goes through periods of being very angry about it, especially when it seems to be disrupting her life or keeping her from reaching her goals. During those times she tinkers with her medication regimen, trying to make the medicine more tolerable to take. When her symptoms get more severe than she can handle on her own, she calls her doctor for help. She has received numerous lectures from doctors over the years for not taking her medications consistently, for waiting until the last minute to call for help, and for not coming to grips with having bipolar disorder. Amanda usually responded to those lectures by changing doctors and repeating the pattern once again.

Amanda had difficulty putting together a Life Chart because there were so many smaller ups and downs between the big episodes of depression and mania.

When she tried to match her medications to her symptoms, she could not remember what she had actually taken or what she had been prescribed. Amanda decided that since she was turning over a new leaf and trying to take charge of her illness she would create a Life Chart that started now and showed her progress in the future. She found a doctor that she liked and made a commitment to herself that she would follow the doctor's instructions for at least the next two years and when she disagreed with him she would talk it over with him.

• **Do periods of excessive drinking or substance abuse about coincide with episodes of depression or mania?** The complicated question is which came first, the mood symptoms or the drinking or drug use? In the section on diagnosis in Chapter 2 is a list of the substances of abuse that can cause symptoms of depression and mania. What we know from research on this topic is that for many people the symptoms of depression or mania came first. If you had not known you had bipolar disorder, you might have looked for ways other than treatment to make yourself feel better. That might have included alcohol or street drugs. Make some notes on your experiences on Worksheet 3.7.

People who have been through this say they started to drink because they couldn't sleep and if they drank enough it would knock them out, or they found that marijuana made it easier to tolerate the agitation and irritability they felt and

---

| worksheet 3.7 | **Alcohol, Drugs, and Symptoms** |

Looking back over your life, can you remember when you started drinking or using street drugs?

Is it possible that you were suffering from depression at the time?

Do you remember feeling less depressed or irritable when you drank or got high?

Could you have been trying to self-medicate?

Overall, how have periods of alcohol or drug use coincided with episodes of depression or mania? Is there an obvious pattern?

could slow their racing thoughts. Tommy swears that he can study more when he smokes pot. Unfortunately, when he gets high regularly, he also forgets to take his medication, and his symptoms of mania return. When this happens, he sees his doctor, gets back into a routine, and his mood stabilizes for a while until he starts smoking regularly again.

Your Treatment History

You have probably discovered that when you see a new doctor or therapist or an old one that you have not seen in a while, he or she wants to know what medications you are taking, why they have changed, and how you are feeling. The typical person who is being treated for bipolar disorder takes several different medications and has usually been through several different trials of other medications. Dosages are changed; medications are stopped and then started again. It can all get very confusing and difficult to remember. The treatment history form in Worksheet 3.8 is a way of keeping track of your medication treatments and their effects. There are places for you to mark what you have been taking, its effect, any side effects it caused, why it was changed, and the doctor who provided it. You can start keeping this log now for your current medications and add to it when changes occur, or you can try to backtrack and fill in the information for previous experiences with medications. You can also keep track of nonpsychiatric medications on this worksheet. Most doctors want to know about all the medications you take. Make extra copies of the blank pages if you need to and take the list with you when you see your doctor or therapist. It will help them understand what you have been through and how to help you and using it will be much less annoying than trying to rely on your memory. An example has been provided on the first line of the form.

➡ *What's Next?*

Now that you have completed your life chart and have begun to identify some patterns, you're on your way to creating a personalized warning system. Remember that one of the most important goals of the CBT approach to the treatment of bipolar disorder is to catch symptoms when they are just beginning to return so that you can take action to keep them from getting worse. The more you know about your history of symptoms, the better prepared you will be to see them coming the next time. In the next chapter you will begin to refine your early warning system by learning ways to track day-to-day changes in mood, thought process, physical symptoms, and behavior. Even if you have had a lot of experience with bipolar disorder and know your symptoms well, it would be a good idea to work through all the exercises in the next chapter.

Your Treatment History

Date	Medication name	Dose and timing	Side effects?	Did it help?	Reason for change	Prescribing doctor
1/1/05	Lithium	300 mg 3 pills in the am and pm	Diarrhea Weight gain	Yes	Depression got worse and gained too much weight	Dr. Smith

(cont.)

From *The Bipolar Workbook* by Monica Ramirez Basco. Copyright 2006 by The Guilford Press. Permission to photocopy this form is granted to purchasers of this book for personal use only (see copyright page for details).

Your Treatment History (*cont.*)

Date	Medication name	Dose and timing	Side effects?	Did it help?	Reason for change	Prescribing doctor

chapter four

Developing
an Early Warning System

In this chapter you will:

✓ Begin to develop a personalized early warning system.
✓ Create a symptom summary worksheet.
✓ Learn to monitor your symptoms using mood graphs.
✓ Learn to recognize the early signs that symptoms are returning.

As you may know, the symptoms of bipolar disorder can come and go throughout your life. There are, however, things you can do to manage severe symptoms and even stop them from recurring. To do this, you must be able to know when the symptoms are beginning to emerge. Having an early warning system can alert you to use CBT methods along with medication to stop the symptoms before they become severe. Whether you were diagnosed recently or you've had the illness for some time, you can benefit from creating an early warning system even if your periods of depression and mania are few and far between.

Know Yourself

The symptoms of depression and mania are obvious and easy to recognize when severe. But usually there are subtle signs that your mood is changing long before it becomes noticeable to others. **The goal is to learn to recognize subtle changes as early as possible.** The quicker you notice them, the quicker you can take action to stop them.

For example, long before you're in a full episode of mania, you might notice more subtle changes. You might become irritable and tense, each day having less and less patience with people. Noises might bother you more and more. And your sleep could slowly worsen from mild insomnia to total sleeplessness.

Symptoms of Mania

Following is a table that lists common symptoms of mania in their mild, moderate, and severe forms. Circle the ones you have experienced.

Common Symptoms of Mania

Mild form of symptom	Moderate form of symptom	Severe manic symptom
Everything seems like a hassle; impatience or anxiety	More easily angered	Irritability
Happier than usual; positive outlook	Increased laughter and joking	Euphoric mood; on top of the world
More talkative; better sense of humor	In the mood to socialize and talk with others	Pressured or rapid speech
More thoughts; mentally sharp, quick; lose focus	Disorganized thinking, poor concentration	Racing thoughts
More self-confident than usual; less pessimistic	Feeling smart, not afraid to try, overly optimistic	Grandiosity—delusions of grandeur
Creative ideas; new interests; change sounds good	Plan to make changes; disorganized in actions, drinking or smoking more	Disorganized activity; starting more things than finishing
Fidgety; nervous behaviors like nail biting	Restless, preferring movement over sedentary activities	Psychomotor agitation; cannot sit still
Not as effective at work; having trouble keeping mind on tasks	Not completing tasks, late for work, annoying others	Cannot complete usual work or home activities
Uncomfortable with other people	Suspicious	Paranoia
More sexually interested	Sexual dreams, seeking out or noticing sexual stimulation	Increased sex drive, seek out sexual activity, more promiscuous
Notice sounds and annoying people; lose train of thought	Noises seem louder, colors seem brighter, mind wanders easily; need quieter environment to focus thoughts	Distractibility—have to work hard to focus thoughts or cannot focus thoughts at all

Symptoms of Depression

You will probably find it easier to recognize the onset of depression than the onset of mania. Long before it's outwardly noticeable to others, you will feel your mood dropping, your attitude becoming more negative, and your desire or interest in activity declining.

For example, before depression might get so severe that you don't want to get out of bed, you could have milder symptoms that suggest you're in for another episode. You might find yourself turning down opportunities to socialize and seeing usual activities as unpleasant or a hassle. Perhaps you'll become more interested in solitary activities, like watching TV or reading. Maybe you would neglect household chores, put less time into your appearance, and slow down in general.

Following is a table that lists common symptoms of depression in their mild, moderate, and severe forms. As you read through, circle the ones that you have experienced in the past.

Common Symptoms of Depression

Mild form of symptom	*Moderate form of symptom*	Severe symptom of depression
Blue, down, or neutral mood	*Cry more easily*	Severe sadness
Not in the mood to socialize	*Less involved with others*	Lack of interest in usual activities
Usual activities are not as much fun as expected	*Have fun until activity is over*	Decreased pleasure
Blame self more readily when things go wrong; see own faults	*Self-critical*	Excessive and inappropriate guilt
Not as hungry as usual; can skip meals occasionally and not feel hungry	*Eating brings less pleasure*	Decreased appetite
Clothes fit slightly looser; no big weight loss (e.g., 1–3 pounds)	*Noticeable weight loss*	Significant weight loss

(cont.)

Common Symptoms of Depression (*cont.*)

Mild form of symptom	Moderate form of symptom	Severe symptom of depression
Sleep seems less restful; ruminating at bedtime; falling asleep takes a little longer	Takes much longer to fall asleep; wake up briefly during the night	Insomnia—cannot fall asleep easily; wake up during the night and stay awake
Lose interest in tasks such as reading; get frustrated with tasks that are lengthy	Must reread text; thoughts cannot be focused well	Impaired concentration
Feel as if you are moving slowly; not mentally sharp	Slowness in movement is noticeable to others; long pauses before answering questions	Psychomotor retardation
Wish pain would go away; thoughts of running away; pessimistic	Thoughts that life may not be worth living; hopeless; can't imagine feeling better	Suicidal ideas or attempts; not caring if you die
Self-doubt; some self-criticism	Low self-esteem; dislike appearance; feel like a loser	Feelings of worthlessness

Your Mood Symptoms

Most people who have been through multiple episodes of depression and mania have difficulty distinguishing symptoms of depression from symptoms of mania. This is because there are some symptoms that are common to both states, such as having trouble sleeping or being irritable. Also when people are having a recurrence of symptoms they just feel bad in general and are fearful of what lies ahead of them. **The reason it is important to know the difference between the onset of mania and the onset of depression is that the treatments you will apply are going to be different.**

The goal of Worksheet 4.1 is to help you begin to distinguish between symptoms of depression and symptoms of mania. This Mood Symptoms Worksheet has three columns for you to fill in—one to describe what you are like when depressed, the second for symptoms of mania, and the third to describe what you are like when you are not having symptoms. Think about each category of symptom and describe how it differs when you are depressed, when you are manic, and when you are feeling OK. For example, what is your mood like when you're depressed? Are you sad or blue? How is it different when you are manic? Do you get happy or irritable? What is your usual mood when you are not having a lot of symptoms? Are you usu-

Mood Symptoms Worksheet

Category	When manic	When depressed	When feeling OK
Mood			
Attitude toward self			
Self-confidence			
Usual activities			
Social activity			
Sleep habits			
Appetite/eating habits			
Concentration			
Speed of thought			
Creativity			
Interest in having fun			
Restlessness			
Sense of humor			
Energy level			
How noise affects you			

(cont.)

Mood Symptoms Worksheet (*cont.*)

Category	When manic	When depressed	When feeling OK
Outlook on the future			
Speech patterns			
Decision-making ability			
Concern for others			
Thoughts about death			
Ability to function			
Other areas:			

ally in a pretty good mood? Are you cranky by nature? Do you feel bored most of the time?

Even for symptoms like insomnia that happen during depression and mania, you can probably tell the difference between these two types of sleeplessness. In depression you may have trouble falling asleep even though you're exhausted. When you wake up in the morning, you're still tired. In mania, you may have too much energy to settle down to fall asleep, and when you wake up in the morning you may feel rested and ready to go.

Try to fill in the Mood Symptoms Worksheet (Worksheet 4.1) with your own examples. You can refer back to the items you circled in the tables of common manic and depressive symptoms. Try to resist writing in "good" or "bad" for each category on the sheet. Instead, try to describe the symptom. For example, under "mood," describe the type of mood you have when you're feeling depressed, (e.g., blue, sad, hopeless, angry, anxious, bored, or miserable). Under the category of sleep, write in how many hours of sleep you get or what kind of trouble you have with your sleep (e.g., can't fall asleep, wake up multiple times, wake up too early and can't go back to sleep).

When you have finished your worksheet, ask your family members or friends to share their observations of the ways they think you change when you're becoming depressed or manic. Add these symptoms to the list. You may not be able to fill in each box today, but as you learn more about yourself in therapy, go back and fill in the symptoms you have begun to notice.

Paul is very familiar with his symptoms. He has read a great deal on the subject and has had the benefit of therapy as well as a good psychiatrist who took a lot of time with Paul and his parents when he was first diagnosed. He attends support group meetings for teenagers and young adults and believes himself to be an expert on the topic. His completed Mood Symptoms Worksheet is provided as an example.

Ways to Use Your Mood Symptoms Worksheet

Suggestion 1

The symptoms you listed are your warning signs that depression or mania may be returning. These are the symptoms to watch for on a regular basis. If you notice any of the warning signs, call your doctor for help and take the precautions you've learned for keeping your symptoms under control.

Suggestion 2

Give a copy of your Mood Symptoms Worksheet to your doctor and therapist. That will help them understand you better and recognize changes in you that you might not notice.

Paul's Worksheet 4.1

Category	When manic	When depressed	When feeling OK
Mood	Irritable	Sad	Content
Attitude toward self	I'm the only one with a brain.	I hate myself.	I'm OK.
Self-confidence	Very self-confident.	No confidence.	I think I am capable of a lot.
Usual activities	Starting but not finishing tasks.	Lie in bed or watch TV.	Work. Clean house. Exercise.
Social activity	Can't stand to be around people.	I don't want anyone to see me.	Visit with friends and family.
Sleep habits	4 hours each night.	Sleep all the time.	7–8 hours of sleep.
Appetite/eating habits	I forget to eat.	I'm not hungry.	I like to eat.
Concentration	Can't hold on to thoughts.	Stare at a page, but can't read.	Pretty good. I can read the paper.
Speed of thought	Fast and disorganized.	My mind is slow and sluggish.	I'm usually a quick thinker.
Creativity	Very creative until I reach my peak.	No creative thoughts.	Can be creative at home.
Interest in having fun	Very interested.	No interest. Nothing is fun.	Some interest.
Restlessness	Very hard to sit still.	I don't want to move off couch.	I like to be busy and keep moving.
Sense of humor	More sarcastic.	Nothing is funny.	Like to tell jokes.
Energy level	High. Nervous energy.	None.	Enough to get things done.
How noise affects you	Noises get on my nerves.	I don't hear what's going on around me.	It doesn't usually bother me.

(cont.)

Category	When manic	When depressed	When feeling OK
Outlook on the future	Anything is possible.	There is no future.	I'm not certain what tomorrow will bring.
Speech patterns	Talk fast and incessantly.	Have difficulty forming words or will not talk.	Talkative, but do not interrupt others.
Decision-making ability	Decisions are made impulsively.	Cannot make decisions.	Can make good decisions.
Concern for others	Not worried about others.	Concerned about what others think of me.	Considerate of others.
Thoughts about death	I think more about God.	Others would be better off without me.	I don't think about it.
Ability to function	At my best for a while.	Can function with a lot of effort.	Function normally.
Other areas: Sex drive	Can't stop thinking about sex.	No interest.	Rarely interested.

Suggestion 3

Give a copy of the worksheet to family members who live with you and can help you monitor your symptoms.

Suggestion 4

If you think you may be having a return of symptoms, but you're not sure, read through the list to see how many symptoms you're having. If you have a few symptoms that are mild, do what you can to keep them from worsening.

Suggestion 5

Here are some questions to ask yourself. If the answer to any is "yes," take action to fix the problem and keep the symptom from worsening.

- *Have I been taking my medication regularly and at the right dose? If not, how do I get back on track?*
- *Have I been getting enough sleep at night? What adjustments do I need to make?*
- *Am I doing anything that could make matters worse? If so, what changes do I need to make?*
- *Are my symptoms getting worse each day? What can I do about it?*
- *Do I need some help? Who should I call?*
- *Is there something I could do today to help myself feel better? Could I change my negative thinking, slow down, get some rest, or take positive actions toward solving a problem?*
- *Should I start monitoring my mood daily?*

If you are uncertain how to make these changes to control symptoms, read ahead to the other chapters for some suggestions. You can also go back and review the table in Chapter 1 called "Where Do I Start?" (pp. 14–15). This table can direct you to specific chapters that might be helpful.

What's Just Me?

If you've struggled with mood swings for many years, you may find it hard to know what is just you and what is the illness. Think of what you're like when you're feeling OK—that is, when not manic or depressed. There are skills, talents, interests, attitudes, and habits that you possess that are unrelated to bipolar disorder. The questions in Worksheet 4.2 on the facing page will help you identify the real you.

Sometimes you may not be aware that you're having symptoms of depression worksheet 4.2 | **The Real You**

What are your usual sleep patterns?

How do you usually spend your time?

How well do you usually manage stress?

Do your feelings get hurt easily?

How well do you get along with others?

Do people usually get on your nerves?

From *The Bipolar Workbook* by Monica Ramirez Basco. Copyright 2006 by The Guilford Press. Permission to photocopy this form is granted to purchasers of this book for personal use only (see copyright page for details).

or mania, but you might notice that you've changed your lifestyle or routine or are not handling life as well as you usually do. For each of the questions you answered in Worksheet 4.2, think about how you might be different when becoming manic or depressed. Make some notes on Worksheet 4.3.

Amanda is still struggling to gain some control over her symptoms. In fact, she has symptoms so often that she's not always sure what normal feels like. She did her best to complete Worksheet 4.3, but she doesn't think there is a distinct difference between how she functions when she is depressed or manic because she tends to have a mix of the two. She knows that she does not function like her old self when she is having mood swings.

You can use this list the same way you use the Mood Symptoms Worksheet (Worksheet 4.1). Review it periodically to determine whether you're acting like your usual self or the way you do when you're getting sick. If you're acting out of the ordinary, make changes by trying to handle things more like your usual self,

| worksheet 4.3 | **Changes You Experience When Symptoms Return** |

	When becoming manic	**When becoming depressed**
What are your usual sleep patterns?		
How do you usually spend your time?		
How well do you usually manage stress?		
Do your feelings get hurt easily?		
How well do you get along with others?		
Do people usually get on your nerves?		

take action to control your symptoms by using the exercises you will be learning in this workbook, and follow your doctor's instructions for controlling symptom breakthroughs with medication.

Monitoring Your Mood

There are several reasons to monitor your mood or other symptoms regularly. The first time you do this exercise, the purpose is to become more tuned in to your daily changes in mood and to find out if there are any specific factors that seem to affect your mood. For example, do you seem to get depressed on rainy days or when you have nothing to do? Do you start to get hyper or manic when there is too much noise or confusion or when you haven't had enough sleep?

You can keep track of mania, hypomania, or depression by monitoring your mood regularly or by watching for other signs or symptoms that mark the beginning of an episode. Some people notice changes in their sleep habits first. Some find it difficult to concentrate. Others find themselves getting more easily annoyed with others.

When he's getting depressed, Paul spends more time in bed. Amanda starts worrying a lot more. Raquel is sentimental and cries when watching TV commercials. When he's getting manic, Tommy is not certain what happens, because he has had bipolar disorder for only a short time, but his friends told him that he wants to party all night when he's manic. His mom says that he picks fights with her. Amanda knows she's getting manic when her house is spotlessly clean.

Amanda's Worksheet 4.3

	When becoming manic	When becoming depressed
What are your usual sleep patterns?	I stay up late.	I go to bed right after dinner but don't fall asleep.
How do you usually spend your time?	I clean the house, catch up on laundry, go to work, go out at night.	I watch television in bed when not at work.
How well do you usually manage stress?	I'm not aware of stress when I'm high.	Poorly. I avoid dealing with things that are stressful.
Do your feelings get hurt easily?	No.	I cry at the smallest thing, think people don't like me.
How well do you get along with others?	I'm the life of the party, the center of attention. I make people laugh.	I get irritated with my family and tend to snap at them. They stay away from me.
Do people get on your nerves?	I can get irritated with stupid people.	Everyone gets on my nerves.

| worksheet 4.4 | **Early Warning Signs of Depression or Mania** |

Look over your answers on the Mood Symptoms Worksheet (Worksheet 4.1) and pick out the symptoms of depression and of mania that you're likely to notice first. Use this worksheet to record these symptoms.

What changes do you notice first when you're getting depressed?

What changes do you notice first when you're getting manic?

Mood Graphs

On pages 73–75 you will find three copies of a Mood Graph (Worksheet 4.5). It's designed so that you can rate your mood each day for one week. The scale in the first column goes from +5 at the top, representing severe mania, to −5 at the bottom, representing severe depression. A rating of 0 in the middle represents a neutral mood, not good or bad.

Each day, circle a dot next to the rating that best describes your mood. At the end of the week, connect the dots to see how your mood has fluctuated. At the bottom of the graph, make notes about any circumstances that might be associated with a change in your mood. Perhaps you forgot to take your medications for a few days, were unable to sleep, or were under a great deal of stress. These clues will help you understand what causes your mood to change and your symptoms to return.

Several copies are included here for your use. You may make additional copies of the Mood Graphs and add them to your workbook as needed.

| **Mood Graph**

Week of:

	Plan	Su	M	T	W	Th	F	Sa
Manic								
+5 Not sleeping, psychotic	*Go to the hospital*	●	●	●	●	●	●	●
+4 Manic, poor judgment		●	●	●	●	●	●	●
+3 Hypomanic	*Call the doctor*	●	●	●	●	●	●	●
+2 Hyper	*Take action*	●	●	●	●	●	●	●
+1 Happy, up	*Watch closely*	●	●	●	●	●	●	●
0 Normal		●	●	●	●	●	●	●
−1 Low, down	*Watch closely*	●	●	●	●	●	●	●
−2 Sad	*Take action*	●	●	●	●	●	●	●
−3 Depressed	*Call the doctor*	●	●	●	●	●	●	●
−4 Immobilized		●	●	●	●	●	●	●
−5 Suicidal	*Go to the hospital*	●	●	●	●	●	●	●
Depressed								

What caused the mood shift?

| **Mood Graph**

Week of:

	Plan	Su	M	T	W	Th	F	Sa
Manic								
+5 Not sleeping, psychotic	Go to the hospital	•	•	•	•	•	•	•
+4 Manic, poor judgment		•	•	•	•	•	•	•
+3 Hypomanic	Call the doctor	•	•	•	•	•	•	•
+2 Hyper	Take action	•	•	•	•	•	•	•
+1 Happy, up	Watch closely	•	•	•	•	•	•	•
0 Normal		•	•	•	•	•	•	•
−1 Low, down	Watch closely	•	•	•	•	•	•	•
−2 Sad	Take action	•	•	•	•	•	•	•
−3 Depressed	Call the doctor	•	•	•	•	•	•	•
−4 Immobilized		•	•	•	•	•	•	•
−5 Suicidal	Go to the hospital	•	•	•	•	•	•	•
Depressed								

What caused the mood shift?

Week of:

	Plan	Su	M	T	W	Th	F	Sa
Manic								
+5 Not sleeping, psychotic	Go to the hospital	●	●	●	●	●	●	●
+4 Manic, poor judgment		●	●	●	●	●	●	●
+3 Hypomanic	Call the doctor	●	●	●	●	●	●	●
+2 Hyper	Take action	●	●	●	●	●	●	●
+1 Happy, up	Watch closely	●	●	●	●	●	●	●
0 Normal		●	●	●	●	●	●	●
−1 Low, down	Watch closely	●	●	●	●	●	●	●
−2 Sad	Take action	●	●	●	●	●	●	●
−3 Depressed	Call the doctor	●	●	●	●	●	●	●
−4 Immobilized		●	●	●	●	●	●	●
−5 Suicidal	Go to the hospital	●	●	●	●	●	●	●
Depressed								

What caused the mood shift?

Symptom Graphs

For some people, it's easier to monitor physical symptoms, sleep habits, or changes in thinking than to monitor mood. Pick a symptom that you would notice changing if you were beginning an episode of depression or mania and write it in on the Symptom Graph (Worksheet 4.6). Here are some common examples:

Monitor changes in *energy level*: +5 means tremendous energy, cannot sit still.
  0 means normal levels of energy.
  −5 means no energy at all, cannot move.

Monitor changes in *concentration*: +5 means so many thoughts you can't speak.
  0 means normal levels of concentration.
  −5 thinking is extremely slow.

Monitor changes in *self-esteem*: +5 means *I think I'm a God.*
  0 means self-esteem is OK.
  −5 means *I hate myself, I have no value.*

After you've picked a symptom, write in a word that would describe what the symptom would look like at each level, from −5 to +5. For example, if you were measuring energy level changes, you might write "tired" next to −2 and "hyper" next to +2. Monitor changes each day and mark them on the graph.

Ways to Use Your Mood and Symptom Graphs

• The primary goal of the Mood Graph is to identify recurrences of symptoms when they are beginning. This can be accomplished by being mindful of mild mood shifts. If you make a habit of rating your mood each day, you will know when changes occur and whether they are reactions to events or more persistent changes that signal a return of symptoms.

• After you've had more experience in tracking your symptoms, you can use these graphs only when you suspect that your symptoms are returning. Monitor your mood or other prominent symptoms daily until they have stabilized.

• The effectiveness of medication changes can be monitored on a mood graph. Begin tracking your mood as medications are added, decreased, or changed to determine the impact on your mood or other symptoms. Make notes on the graph as doses are changed to help you and your doctor monitor their effect.

• Mood Graphs are helpful for communicating to your doctor how you have been doing between visits, especially if they are separated by several weeks. Track your mood daily and make notes on the graph about any circumstances you associate with improvements or worsening of your mood. This will help you and your

| **Symptom Graph**

Week of:									
	Plan	**Day 1**	**Day 2**	**Day 3**	**Day 4**	**Day 5**	**Day 6**	**Day 7**
Manic									
+5	*Go to the hospital*	●	●	●	●	●	●	●
+4		●	●	●	●	●	●	●
+3	*Call the doctor*	●	●	●	●	●	●	●
+2	*Take action*	●	●	●	●	●	●	●
+1	*Watch closely*	●	●	●	●	●	●	●
0		●	●	●	●	●	●	●
−1	*Watch closely*	●	●	●	●	●	●	●
−2	*Take action*	●	●	●	●	●	●	●
−3	*Call the doctor*	●	●	●	●	●	●	●
−4		●	●	●	●	●	●	●
−5	*Go to the hospital*	●	●	●	●	●	●	●
Depressed									

What caused the change?

health care provider better understand your symptom fluctuations and what can be done to minimize the ones that are extreme or persistent.

• When you begin seeing a new doctor or therapist, you can help him or her get to know you and the pattern of your symptoms by monitoring your mood and taking the graphs to each visit. This will make it easier for you to communicate what happens between visits rather than having to rely solely on your memory.

What's Next?

If you have worked through all the exercises in this chapter, your early warning system is now complete. The next step is to put your monitoring plan into action. Practice what you've learned by using the Mood Graph and the Mood Symptoms Worksheet on a regular basis. Because it's easy to get busy and forget to monitor your symptoms, some people put a reminder note to themselves in their workspace, on their refrigerator, or on their bathroom mirror. If privacy is not a problem, it's best to put your worksheet in a place that you can see every day.

It's time to go to Step 2 and learn how to take precautions to avoid relapse. In the next chapter you will learn about the various things that can make mania and depression worse and how to avoid them. Even people who have had a lot of experience with bipolar disorder find these guidelines helpful. Take the next step in learning how to prevent depression and mania from coming back.

Step 2

Take Precautions

chapter five

Making Yourself Less Vulnerable

> *In this chapter you will:*
>
> ✓ Learn what behaviors can make mania and depression worse.
> ✓ Find ways to increase contact with and support from others.
> ✓ Make improvements in your eating and sleeping habits.
> ✓ Control worry and rumination.
> ✓ Reduce overstimulation.
> ✓ Stop procrastination.
> ✓ Make overwhelming tasks more manageable.

This chapter is divided into three parts: (1) how not to make it worse once symptoms begin, (2) how to increase the positives in your life, and (3) how to decrease and control the negatives. If you are newly diagnosed, you probably haven't had enough experience with the illness to know the kinds of things that can make depression and mania worse or better. Reading this chapter can make you aware of the kinds of problems you might encounter as well as some protections you can put in place to make your life better. You will also want to reread this chapter from time to time when you do encounter symptoms and are not sure how to cope.

Those who are highly experienced with the illness but still struggle to gain and maintain control over symptoms will want to work carefully through each of the exercises in this chapter. These exercises are particularly suited for you.

If you feel like your illness is fairly stable, you'll probably find that you already do many of the things recommended here. If so, you may want to use the exercises in this chapter when you're having a recurrence of symptoms as a reminder of how to regain control.

How *Not* to Make It Worse

In the first chapter of this workbook, the cognitive–behavioral model of bipolar disorder was explained. Now it's time to put that model to work.

The Course of Bipolar Disorder

When you suffer from depression, mania, hypomania, or mixed states, you undergo changes in your mood, your thinking patterns, your actions, and your physical functioning. These changes seem to build on one another, creating more and more distress. To refresh your memory, the diagram labeled "Course of Bipolar Disorder" shows how an episode of depression or mania can lead to changes in your thoughts and your mood.

Sad moods are usually accompanied by negative thoughts about yourself, your world, and your future. Euphoric moods bring about optimistic thoughts, a more positive self-view, and ideas for new activities or adventures. Irritable moods can stimulate negative thoughts about other people and suspiciousness. Changes in your thoughts and your feelings will affect your behavior. When feeling depressed and thinking poorly about yourself, you will slow down or become less active. The more your mood worsens and the more negative your attitude becomes, the less active you will be at home, at work, and in socializing with other people. You will natu-

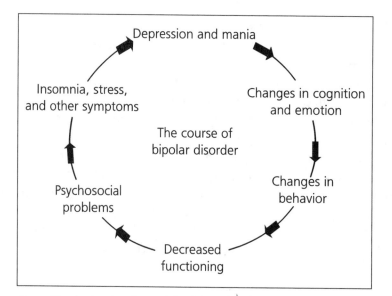

Cognitive-behavioral model of bipolar disorder.

rally feel an urge to pull back or withdraw from others, not wanting to be bothered. On Worksheet 5.1, make some notes about the ways your behavior changes when you're getting depressed.

When you're beginning an episode of mania, your changes in behavior might not be obvious to you, but they are usually noticeable to others, especially those who know you well. Whether your mood has become more euphoric or more irritable, there is often an increase in activity. This might include restlessness, moving around more than usual, changing frequently from one activity to another, or taking more risks. When mania is mild, many people feel a desire to pursue more activities or make changes in their usual routine, but they may resist the urge, forcing themselves to finish a task that they've started. On Worksheet 5.2, make some notes about the changes in behavior you experience when manic.

---

worksheet 5.1 | **Behavior Changes in Depression**

When I am depressed I have noticed that my behavior changes in the following ways:

_____   _____

_____   _____

_____   _____

_____   _____

---

worksheet 5.2 | **Behavior Changes in Mania**

When I am becoming more manic, I have noticed the following changes in my behavior:

_____   _____

_____   _____

_____   _____

_____   _____

The changes in your thoughts, feelings, and actions during episodes of depression and mania can begin to interfere with your life if they keep you from following your usual routine or from meeting your responsibilities. Once your day-to-day functioning begins to decline, it doesn't take long for bigger problems to emerge. Having problems can keep you up at night and cause you a great deal of stress, which, in turn, worsens your symptoms of depression or mania.

The goal of this workbook is to teach you skills for breaking this cycle so that the changes in your thoughts, feelings, and behaviors can return to normal before they interfere with your ability to function, create big problems, and worsen your stress.

How Not to Make It Worse

Just as there are many things you can do to make yourself feel better, there are always things that can make your symptoms worse. In addition to learning new strategies for improving your symptoms of depression or mania, try to control the factors that are likely to make matters worse. The plan will probably be different for depression than for mania.

What Makes Depression Worse?

The answer to this question is probably different for each person with bipolar disorder. However, many people find that stress, inactivity, withdrawing from others, and getting angry with themselves always seem to compound their misery.

Feeling Overwhelmed

Problems with work, family members, or your physical health can occur unpredictably. If you're already depressed, it's easy to get overly stressed when you find you have a new problem to overcome. In fact, even if the problem is manageable, it's not unusual to become so overwhelmed when thinking about all you must accomplish that your coping abilities fail you. In this case, it's not just that you have a problem that worsens your depression. It's the fact that in your mind it becomes overwhelming, unmanageable, and further evidence that your life is bad. To avoid making matters worse, you have to try not to clump all of your problems into one big disaster. You have to try to see each problem individually, solving one at a time or getting assistance from others to solve one at a time. Later in this chapter are some instructions for doing this.

Isolation from Others

Although your instinct when depressed might be to pull away or isolate yourself from others, it's probably one of the worst things you can do. You need the benefits of interacting with others. When you're alone, it's easy to ruminate more, allow yourself to slack off on personal hygiene, and end up missing out on the positive aspects of being around other people. There's no one to talk to about your problems, no one to make you laugh or take your mind off your worries, and no one to give you encouragement and hope. The obvious solution is to make yourself have contact with family members, friends, coworkers, or other people in your world. Make phone calls, accept offers to meet with people, eat your meals with the family, and go to work so that you can be around positive people. Forcing yourself to make these efforts isn't always easy when you're depressed, of course, so this chapter provides some ideas for getting you back into contact with others. Chapters 8 and 9 offer exercises for controlling the negative thoughts that might talk you out of interacting with people.

Anger

If you have been through periods of depression in the past, it's easy to get angry with yourself when symptoms return. But getting angry about being depressed only makes you feel worse. Getting depressed about the fact that you're going through another episode of depression compounds your misery, making it harder to bring yourself out of the episode. It's OK to be angry about having bipolar disorder and being forced to go through another round of depression. You have the right to be mad, frustrated, or disappointed. However, it's best to acknowledge your annoyance and then let it go long enough to work at pulling yourself through it. Staying mad only fuels the fire. The exercises in this chapter help you work around your anger. In Chapter 7 anger over having bipolar disorder will be discussed specifically.

Negative Input

Movies with tragic themes or plots, sad songs, other people's problems, thinking about the past, television news, and people with negative attitudes, words, facial expressions, and actions can all worsen depression.

Many other things can worsen a depression. Take a moment and write down on Worksheet 5.3 things that you know will worsen your depression. Consider how certain people can make you feel worse, as can changes in routine, self-destructive behaviors, or not taking any positive action. These are the things you should avoid when you think your symptoms of depression are returning.

| worksheet 5.3 | **Things That Make Depression Worse** |

Things that can make my depression worse	What I am going to do about it

Amanda's Worksheet 5.3

Things that can make my depression worse	What I am going to do about it
Thinking about the past.	Cook a meal to distract myself.
Listing my faults and failures.	Think about my children.
Watching sad movies on TV.	Get out of bed, turn off TV, and do something in another room.
Getting "advice" from my mom.	Screen my calls. Call her when I'm feeling better.
Drinking wine.	Go to an extra AA meeting if I need it.

What Makes Mania Worse?

Among the most common factors that worsen mania are losing sleep, getting over-stimulated, missing doses of medication, using stimulant drugs or alcohol, and trying to stay on a high.

Staying High

The enjoyment of the high before it gets out of control is the reason some people push themselves to extend it. Their hope is to stay hypomanic without letting it become a full episode of mania. Unfortunately, it rarely works out that way. Hypomania usually evolves into mania, and mania is often followed by a severe drop into depression. Although most people would say that in the long run it's not worth the risk, trying to ride out the high is still one of the common things that people do that inevitably makes matters worse. In Chapter 10, strategies will be covered for making good decisions about staying high versus controlling your symptoms. In Chapter 7, you will have a chance to explore your feelings about taking control of your illness. The exercises provided in those chapters will help you avoid making yourself feel worse when you see mania coming on.

Losing Sleep

Losing the ability to sleep is a symptom of hypomania and mania, but it is also what seems to make the problem worse. Studies on sleep patterns in mood disorders have shown that loss of sleep can push a person with bipolar disorder into mania. Sleep loss can be caused by travel, thinking about problems at bedtime, working overtime, hearing disturbing noises at night, or getting too involved in fun activities around bedtime. Losing sleep for these reasons can quickly turn into insomnia, in which you can't fall asleep. Most sleep researchers suggest going to bed and waking up at about the same time each day. To prevent your symptoms from worsening, follow these simple rules: Avoid all-nighters, schedule travel to ensure a good night's sleep, and work out your worries before you go to bed. In the remaining sections of this chapter you will learn how.

Skipping Medication

Not taking medication can definitely make things worse. Issues about taking medication are covered in the next chapter. If you're not convinced that you need to stay on medication or if you think your regimen needs to change, talk it over with your doctor before you take any action. Remember that the symptoms of bipolar disorder can alter your thinking and make you feel discouraged about taking medication. Chapter 6 will give you some ideas for getting the most out of your medication treatment.

Overstimulation

Too much noise, confusion, light, activity, and change can cause overstimulation. Dealing with these sources of overstimulation will be covered in the third major part of this chapter. For now, write down your thoughts about what can make your mania worse on Worksheet 5.4.

It has been a long time since Raquel has had a full manic episode, but she does get mildly manic or hypomanic from time to time. On the facing page are her ideas for keeping her manic symptoms from worsening when they appear.

| worksheet 5.4 | **Things That Can Make Mania Worse** |

Things that can make my mania worse	What I am going to do about it

Raquel's Worksheet 5.4

Things that can make my mania worse	What I am going to do about it
Shopping in malls, especially during big sales.	Avoid them when manic or limit shopping to only necessities.
Surfing the Internet late at night.	Check e-mail in the morning or get online right after dinner.
Family gatherings. Too many people and too much noise.	When overstimulated, go into a quiet room for a while or leave early.

Increasing Positives

When you're trying to make changes in your life and control your mood swings, it's much easier to add positives than to take away negatives. For example, picking up a new healthy habit and adding it to your routine can always be accomplished more easily than breaking a bad habit. After you have mastered the previous section and learned how not to make matters worse, focus your attention on trying to increase positives in your life. That includes positive people, positive experiences, improved sleep, and developing healthy habits.

Adding People

When you get depressed, you may not feel like being around others. It may seem like too much hassle, people might seem annoying or uncaring, or you might not want them to know what's going on with you. Perhaps you feel anxious about how you'll act or how others will treat you. Although keeping to yourself is a natural urge, it is probably one of the worst things you can do when depressed. Isolation breeds loneliness. Loneliness fuels depression. Depression makes you want to isolate yourself even more. It can become a vicious cycle. While you are alone you have too much time to dwell on your misery, you have no one to talk you out of your negative thinking, and you miss opportunities to laugh. In spite of the fact that family members or friends do not always say the right things, you need them for support or at least for a distraction from your pain.

Depression

⮕ ⮕ ⮕ leads to **Isolation**

⮕ ⮕ ⮕ which leads to **Loneliness**

⮕ ⮕ ⮕ which leads to more **Depression**

The solution is to do the opposite of what you feel like doing. Instead of pulling away from people, move toward them. Let people know you're feeling down. Call on a friend, a family member, someone from your place of worship, a support group member, a coworker, your therapist or doctor, or a neighbor. Don't hide. Let people reach out to you and offer their aid. They may not be able to solve your problems, but they can stand by your side to give you the added strength you might need to solve your own problems.

Psyching Yourself Up for Socializing

To talk yourself into socializing when your instinct tells you to stay away, you have to think of reasons it can be good to interact with others. Think of past experiences when being around other people felt good or was helpful in some way. Perhaps repeating these types of interactions would motivate you to do more. On Worksheet 5.5, record the positives you've derived from interacting with people in the past, which are good reasons to interact in the present.

Adding Healthy Habits

On Worksheet 5.6, list the healthy habits you already have and those you would like to develop or strengthen. Include better ways to manage your symptoms, organize your life, and get more enjoyment out of life.

| worksheet 5.5 | **Good Reasons to Interact with People** |

When I have contact with people, I get these positives out of it:

From *The Bipolar Workbook* by Monica Ramirez Basco. Copyright 2006 by The Guilford Press. Permission to photocopy this form is granted to purchasers of this book for personal use only (see copyright page for details).

Paul's Worksheet 5.5

When I have contact with people, I get these positives out of it:

I temporarily forget about my problems.

They can make me laugh.

I can get out of myself for a little while.

Afterward I'm always glad I did it.

Amanda's Worksheet 5.5

When I have contact with people, I get these positives out of it:

They remind me that I do have support if I want it.

I get a reality check from my overly negative thinking. My family tells me I'm not as worthless as I think and I'm not alone in my misery.

Going to church with others gives me hope.

---

worksheet 5.6 | **Healthy Habits**

Healthy habits I regularly practice:

_____

_____

_____

Healthy habits I need to strengthen:

_____

_____

_____

New healthy habits I would like to develop:

_____

_____

_____

Healthy habits I used to have and would like to restart:

_____

_____

_____

Tommy's Worksheet 5.6

Healthy habits I regularly practice:

I exercise pretty often.

I avoid eating French fries/chips.

Healthy habits I need to strengthen:

Getting up on time for school.

Getting to bed sooner.

New healthy habits I would like to develop:

Reading more.

Drinking less often.

Stop getting speeding tickets.

Healthy habits I used to have and would like to restart:

Eating healthily.

Getting all my homework done.

Going to every class.

Weight Control

Weight gain is one of the more common complaints of people who take medications for bipolar disorder. Not all the blame can be placed on medications, however. It's easy to develop poor eating habits and to put off regular exercise. Medications may make you crave unhealthy foods, and depression can make you seek out pleasure from food. But once you start eating high-fat or high-sugar foods and neglecting the healthier options, it's easy to get hooked on them. Some people try to justify their bad eating habits by saying that since they have to suffer with bipolar disorder, they have the right to enjoy the foods they like. Others say that eating is the only pleasure they have in life. Neither of these ideas would be so bad if pleasure foods didn't make you gain weight.

It may be a good idea to diet and exercise, but many people put it off. When told by their doctors to start a diet program or exercise plan, they might initially resist, raising objections like those listed on Worksheet 5.7. Circle the ones that apply to you.

It's true that changing your eating habits can be a big challenge and exercise can be hard to do. But most people want to get in better shape so that they can do more and feel better about themselves. If you follow the logic that it's easier to add a positive than take away a negative, you can make positive changes to your eating habits and activity that might help you control your weight. Start with one positive habit until you have mastered it and then add another. When you feel more confident that you can make changes, start eliminating negatives. The table on the facing page lists some examples of positives you can add that will help you work toward healthier dietary and activity habits. As you read through the list, think about the ones you might be able to do.

If you think improving your eating habits and exercise is more than you can handle, skip ahead to the section later in this chapter called "Feeling Overwhelmed" and use the exercise for breaking down the task before taking it on. It will help you figure out where to start.

Once you've added some healthy habits, you may be ready to eliminate a few unhealthy ones. Worksheet 5.8 contains a list of negative habits you might consider eliminating. Try to make a change in one and master it before adding another.

It's easy to think of diet programs in an all-or-nothing way: You either have to do it all—make all the positive changes, deny yourself "bad" foods, eat on a consis-

---

worksheet 5.7 | **Weight Control Obstacles**

- I don't know how to diet.
- I hate to exercise.
- I can't handle a diet right now.
- I don't want to diet.
- It will stress me out too much.

- I don't have money for diet foods.
- I can't afford a gym membership.
- It shouldn't matter that I'm fat.
- I've tried and I can't do it.
- I like sweets.

Add These Positives to Control Weight and Get Fit

- Read a book on dieting.
- Join Weight Watchers.
- Read the nutritional labels on foods.
- Choose items that are healthier for you.
- Add a piece of fruit to your lunch.
- Find a vegetable that you like to eat.
- Cook meals more often.

- Go for a walk every day.
- Scrub floors, mow the lawn, rake leaves.
- Watch an exercise show on TV and try to follow along.
- Walk your dog farther than usual.
- Wear a pedometer.
- Play with a young child.

tent schedule, totally work the program—or not do it at all. Coping with bipolar disorder is hard enough. Trying to follow a diet program 100% of the time may get you the best results, but if it's too difficult, you won't stick with it. Worksheet 5.9 includes some general ideas that may help you improve your eating habits. Put a check (✓) next to the ones you already do and two checks (✓✓) next to the ones you want to try.

| worksheet 5.8 | **Eliminating Negatives to Control Weight and Get Fit** |

Put a check next to the ones that might be right for you.

- Do not keep junk food at home. If you want a treat, go out and buy one serving. If it is at your fingertips, it will be harder to resist.

- Look through your grocery cart before you check out. Count how many items you are about to buy that would be considered unhealthy. If there are several, take some out. The clerk will be happy to reshelve them for you.

- Try to go without sweets for a few days until your cravings decrease.

- Trade out full-sugar soft drinks for diet drinks or water.

- Try to eat a meal without adding bread.

- Eat grilled instead of fried foods.

- Count how many sweets you eat in a day and challenge yourself to reduce them by half.

| worksheet 5.9 | **Ways to Improve Your Eating Habits** |

- Think before you eat. Make choices that are better for you.

- Use your resources. You don't have to do this alone. Ask for help.

- Join a group of people who are working toward the same goal.

- Do the best you can as often as you can rather than approaching it in an all-or-nothing way.

- Set a series of small personal goals instead of a large weight-loss goal.

- Remember that one meal or one day of poor eating does not blow the whole plan. Just make a commitment to yourself to do better the next day.

- Weight loss takes time. Don't expect overnight changes and then feel discouraged if they don't come right away.

- Before you buy foods labeled *low-fat,* read the label and compare the calorie count and carbohydrate content to those of the regular version.

- Ask yourself how hungry you really are before you eat. If you're just bored and not hungry, do something else. If you're upset and not really hungry at all, use one of the other methods in this workbook to help you feel better. If you're just thirsty, drink something and reevaluate your hunger afterward. If you *are* hungry, eat an amount that matches the amount of hunger you feel. Sometimes a small amount of food will do the trick. Remember, you can save the rest for later.

Getting a Good Night's Sleep

Another positive to add to your life is to get enough sleep. The table at the top of the facing page lists strategies you can use to ensure a good night's sleep. If you're doing all you can to sleep well and still have insomnia, talk to your doctor about sleep aids.

What If I Can't Fall Asleep?

Just as there are things you can do to help yourself get a good night's sleep, there are a number of things you probably should *not* do. Things that can interfere with a good night's sleep are listed in the table at the bottom of the facing page.

Tips for a Good Night's Sleep

- *Be consistent.* Try to go to bed and wake up at about the same time each day, even on weekends.

- *It's a nighttime thing.* Avoid sleeping during the day and staying awake late at night. If your sleep cycle is already switched around, work with your doctor on a plan for getting your sleep back to normal.

- *Keep your bed as a place for sleep.* Make it a habit to watch TV, eat, read, or pay your bills in another room, at a table, or on a couch. Teach your body to associate going to bed with falling asleep.

- *Get comfortable.* Make your sleep area comfortable by picking pillows, blankets, and clothing that make you feel good.

- *Gear down for the night.* Start preparing to sleep at least an hour ahead of time by quieting your environment and quieting your mind.

- *Avoid stimulants that might keep you awake.* A hot cup of cocoa or coffee, a few cigarettes, or some dessert might sound good at nighttime, but for those who are sensitive to caffeine, nicotine, or sugar, they may make it harder to fall asleep. If you have any digestive problems, late dinners or spicy meals might trouble your stomach and keep you awake.

Things *Not* to Do When You Are Having Trouble Sleeping

- *Caffeine.* Don't make yourself a pot of coffee. The caffeine can keep you awake. If you enjoy a hot cup of coffee on a cold night, buy some decaffeinated coffee for evening and nighttime use.

- *Internet.* Avoid getting out of bed to surf the Internet. Instead of getting sleepy, you will most likely stimulate your brain and keep yourself awake.

- *TV and books.* If you are going to watch television or read a book, choose something that is not likely to keep you awake. A good boring book or a television rerun will do the trick. Avoid shows with people arguing, cliffhangers, violence, or real-life docudramas.

- *Chores.* Don't get up and clean your house. Although unfinished chores may be on your mind, the process of doing physical labor in the middle of the night will tense your muscles rather than relax them. To be mentally alert enough to do chores you have to stay awake. This defeats the purpose of getting a good night's sleep.

- *Exercise.* It is probably not a good idea to get out of bed to exercise even if you know that exercise can wear you out. Physical activity can overstimulate your mind and body. If exercise is usually a good idea for you, schedule time before you go to bed to work out.

Don't Panic

Anxiety and sleep are not a good mix. Starting to worry or even panic about your inability to sleep will only make it harder to fall asleep. Sleep happens automatically. It is not a thing you can easily will your body to do, so the harder you work at convincing yourself to fall asleep, the longer it can take. Not being able to fall asleep can also leave you frustrated and even aggravated. Strong emotions like this are not conducive to falling asleep.

Calm Your Body

Your body and your mind work together to help you fall asleep. If your mind is too busy to settle down, you can help the process along by trying to relax your body. Start with your toes and work toward your head. Focus on letting go of tensions in each muscle and getting your body into a comfortable position. Work on one foot at a time, then one leg at a time, and so on. Make sure you relax the muscles in your face, especially your forehead, jaw, and eyes. After you have relaxed from head to toe, count to ten slowly and with each number try to let go and relax just a little bit more. Search for any remaining tension and release it. If you like this kind of strategy, you may want to try the more elaborate relaxation exercise provided in Chapter 10.

Too Alert to Fall Asleep?

If you're too wide awake to fall asleep, you would be better off getting out of bed and doing something else relaxing, like watching television, reading a book, or any other activity that usually calms you or tires your mind.

Decreasing Negatives

Now that you have figured out how not to make matters worse when your symptoms begin and you have created a plan for adding positives to your life, it's time to focus your attention on eliminating negatives. This section provides instructions and suggestions for reducing worry and rumination, coping with overstimulation, overcoming lethargy, and controlling manic urges for change and activity.

Nighttime Worry and Rumination

As you begin to relax your body to fall asleep, sometimes your mind will wander over the events of the day, conversations with other people, or problems that you face. It seems involuntary. The thoughts just pop into your head, and one idea can lead to another. Pretty soon you can find yourself more mentally alert than before you went to bed. If you frequently have this kind of bedtime experience, it's time to try something new. Here are the steps to control nighttime worry and rumination.

- **Step 1: Make time to review your day,** your worries, and your problems before you go to bed, preferably more than an hour before bedtime. Raquel liked to set aside time before the evening news. Watching the news made it easier for her to let go of her day and get ready for bed.
- **Step 2: Make a list.** As you begin to think about the things that bother you, write them down. If you see them in writing, you won't need to keep them in your head. Here is one of Raquel's lists:

Raquel's Daily Review List

I got up too late.
The boss was in a bad mood.
The dog didn't eat all his food today.
My skirt felt too tight. I'm gaining weight again.
Pick up the dry cleaning for husband.
Call Mom this weekend and try to cheer her up.
Don't forget to return the DVDs from the video store.

- **Step 3: Prioritize.** Try to put the items on your list in some sort of order according to their importance. Little things can sometimes feel like they have great importance because they happened most recently or because they were really annoying. Make the order of worries reflect the significance of items in the grand scheme of your life. Here is how Raquel prioritized her list.

(1) I got up too late.
(9) The boss was in a bad mood.
(6) The dog didn't eat all his food today.
(5) My skirt felt too tight. I'm gaining weight again.
(8) Pick up the dry cleaning for husband.
(7) Call Mom this weekend and try to cheer her up.
(10) Don't forget to return the DVDs from the video store.

She skipped numbers 2–4 and made her second item a ranking of 5 to remind herself that the next most important item is not very important in the grand scheme of things. Getting up on time was important because it made the rest of her day go more smoothly. The other items, 5 to 10, were not all that important to Raquel and certainly were not worth losing sleep over.

- **Step 4: Make a plan of action** for the items that bother you the most. Think of something you can do tomorrow to take a step toward its solution even if it means you will only schedule time to think about it more, talk to someone about it, or get more information on the subject. You don't have to feel burdened with resolving big issues all at once. Think about a logical first step by considering your options and select one that might help you achieve your goals. Write down your plan so that you will not have to hold it in your memory. Raquel wrote down a few ideas for the items she thought she could control.

> *(1) I got up too late. Set the alarm clock for 15 minutes earlier.*
> *(9) The boss was in a bad mood. Nothing I can do.*
> *(6) The dog didn't eat all his food today. Talk to kids about not giving him snacks.*
> *(5) My skirt felt too tight. I need to stay away from bread for a while.*
> *(8) Pick up the dry cleaning for husband. Tell him to do it.*
> *(7) Call Mom this weekend and try to cheer her up. I may not be able to make her feel better.*
> *(10) Don't forget to return the DVDs from the video store. Put them in the car before I forget.*

- **Step 5: Stop the thought.** If what you are ruminating about is not very important or is beyond your control, but keeps popping into your head, tell yourself to "Stop." Use a forceful tone with yourself, even if it's only in your thoughts. Remind yourself that rumination is a waste of your energy. Refocus your thoughts and energy on something worthwhile or within your realm of control. If that doesn't work, try switching your thought to something more pleasant, like remembering a walk in the park or the last time you saw a beautiful sunset.

Overstimulation

There are two sources of stimulation that can make mania and hypomania worse. The first group includes stimulation from your environment, such as noise, and the second is internal stimulation that comes from having a lot of thoughts or ideas. Too much external stimulation can make you feel irritable or anxious. It can worsen racing thoughts and make it hard for you to concentrate. Overstimulation can keep you awake at night. Even positive things such as people laughing and having fun can be mentally overstimulating at times. Things in your environment that can overstimulate you are listed in the table at the top of the facing page.

Sometimes your own thoughts and activities can be overstimulating. For exam-

Sources of Overstimulation in Your Environment

- Noise
- Clutter
- Confusion
- Too many people
- Traffic on the road

- Loud laughter
- Loud music
- Phones ringing
- Children playing
- Group therapy

ple, if you're beginning to have symptoms of mania or hypomania, you might have more ideas than usual and you might be more creative as well. The more you think about your new ideas, the more stimulated you become. Emotions such as joy or excitement may seem to escalate the process, especially if you try to put your ideas into action. The more excited you get, the faster your ideas will flow. This might actually feel good until you become overly stimulated, have more thoughts than you can handle, and begin to feel agitated or exhausted. Unfortunately, it's hard to stop the process when it has gone on too long. Examples of things that can overstimulate you are listed in the table below.

Reducing Environmental Stimulation

The first step in reducing overstimulation is to **recognize** that it is occurring. You might be aware of feeling uptight, anxious, or unsettled, but you might not always recognize its source. Amanda can feel herself tightening up when the kids are running around the house and screaming. The second step is to **identify** the source of stimulation. Is it something in your environment or something within you? In Amanda's case it's her kids. The third step is to **take action.** Amanda can redirect

Examples of Internal Overstimulation

- Racing thoughts
- Rumination about the past
- Making plans for new activities or adventures
- Mulling over creative thoughts or ideas
- Repeating thoughts to store in memory instead of writing them down
- Starting new projects
- Reminiscing about the past, especially emotional events

the kids' activities so that they do something less noisy, or she can leave the room until she feels more able to handle it.

If the source of stimulation is something in your environment, find a way to quiet it down or distance yourself from it. This might mean lowering the volume on the television or radio, walking away from a crowd of people, or asking children to play more quietly. Find a quiet place to gather your thoughts and calm yourself. You can go to another room, take a quiet walk, turn out the lights and lie down, or sit in your car for a while.

If a cluttered environment is the source of overstimulation, you can leave it or you can try to fix it. To fix it, read ahead to the section "Feeling Overwhelmed" (p. 106). Apply the step-by-step procedure for gaining control over your environment by fixing one thing at a time.

Reducing Internal Stimulation

In many ways it's easier to control external stimulation than it is to control internal stimulation. You can walk away from a busy environment, but you can't easily walk away from a busy mind. To reduce internal stimulation you have to find a way to quiet your mind or organize your thoughts. The goal is to slow your mental processes so they are no longer overstimulating. Here are some ideas:

• **Get quiet.** Taking action to quiet your environment is a good first step. If there is less noise on the outside, there will be less confusion in your head. Follow the instructions in the previous section for reducing external stimulation.

• **Calm yourself.** Mental overstimulation seems to be fueled by strong emotions such as anxiety or excitement. Use a relaxation exercise to reduce tension in your body, distract yourself for a while with soothing music, or put your feet up and rest for a short while. Anything you've found in the past to be relaxing or that has helped you wind down when you were stressed can usually reduce mental overstimulation.

• **Get organized.** One of the symptoms of hypomania and mania is having an increased number of ideas for new activities or adventures. Sometimes you feel a surge of motivation that makes you want to take care of neglected chores, begin a creative task, or make a change in some aspect of your life. It may seem like one new idea just leads to another. This can feel good, especially if you've been suffering from depression recently and your thoughts have been slow or your motivation has been low. But if you don't set a limit on internal stimulation, it can reach a point where you have too many ideas and your thoughts become disorganized and distressing. To control the urge to follow each new idea when it comes to mind, try the following goal-setting exercise to get organized.

Goal Setting

When you feel yourself getting overstimulated or overwhelmed by too many ideas or too much to do, use Worksheet 5.10 to help you organize your thoughts. When mania and hypomania begin to emerge, all new ideas might seem like they are high priority. You might go from one project to another, starting many but finishing few. Each activity might seem like a reasonable thing to do, but if you try to do too much, you'll overstimulate yourself in the process.

Use the Goal-Setting Worksheet to write down all the activity ideas that come to mind. This would include things you have to do, things you want to do, and things you've been putting off for some time. Once you have them all written down, try to determine whether each item is a high (**H**), medium (**M**), or low (**L**) priority. There is a column with H, M, and L next to each item. Circle the one that applies. *High priority* can mean that the task is something very important or that has an immediate deadline. High-priority tasks might include paying your rent or getting your medication refilled. *Low-priority* tasks are those that can wait. There is no consequence if they don't get done right away, like watching a particular movie or reorganizing your closet. Low-priority tasks also include things that have only a small consequence if not completed, for example, going to the grocery store to buy more milk. In this case you would like to do it if you had time, but it's not an emergency. *Medium-priority* tasks are somewhere in the middle between high- and low-priority tasks.

When you are finished with your list and have made your priority ratings, review the list. If you have too many items marked as high priorities, reconsider whether these are things that absolutely must be done right away or could wait until you have more time. On the first pass, it's easy to think that everything is a high priority even when it is not.

For the items that really are high priorities, put them in order of how you want to complete them, with *1* next to the most important and highest-priority item, *2* next to the second-most-important item, and so on. Put these numbers in the column labeled "Rank Order."

Next comes the hard part. You have to make yourself do one thing at a time, starting with the highest-priority item. Even though your instinct may be to jump from one activity to another, make a deal with yourself to finish one task before going on to the next.

| **Goal-Setting Worksheet**

Current activities, responsibilities, and interests	Priority			Rank order
	High	**Medium**	**Low**	
_____	H	M	L	_____
_____	H	M	L	_____
_____	H	M	L	_____
_____	H	M	L	_____
_____	H	M	L	_____
_____	H	M	L	_____
_____	H	M	L	_____
_____	H	M	L	_____
_____	H	M	L	_____
_____	H	M	L	_____
_____	H	M	L	_____
_____	H	M	L	_____
_____	H	M	L	_____
_____	H	M	L	_____
_____	H	M	L	_____
_____	H	M	L	_____
_____	H	M	L	_____
_____	H	M	L	_____
_____	H	M	L	_____

Paul's Worksheet 5.10

Current activities, responsibilities, and interests	Priority			Rank order
	High	**Medium**	**Low**	
Finish reading new book	H	M	Ⓛ	
Pay the rent	Ⓗ	M	L	_1_
Return Mom's call	H	Ⓜ	L	
Get oil changed in car	H	Ⓜ	L	
Ask Alice out for Friday night	Ⓗ	M	L	_3_
Make a bank deposit	H	Ⓜ	L	
Figure out codes on PS2 game	H	M	Ⓛ	
Apply for a job	H	Ⓜ	L	
Take in computer to be repaired	Ⓗ	M	L	_7_
Buy groceries	H	Ⓜ	L	
Buy cigars	Ⓗ	M	L	_8_
Refill med prescription	H	Ⓜ	L	
Do laundry—underwear	Ⓗ	M	L	_4_
Go to class	H	Ⓜ	L	
Fix broken window on car	Ⓗ	M	L	_5_
Get Alice's phone number	Ⓗ	M	L	_2_
Finish writing paper for class	Ⓗ	M	L	_6_
	H	M	L	
	H	M	L	

Feeling Overwhelmed

- Do you know exactly what to do, but can't make yourself do it?
- When you begin to face a difficult task, do you immediately think about all the parts that need to be accomplished and feel exhausted and discouraged before you even start?
- Does it seem like more than you can handle right how?
- Does this make you procrastinate and put things off much longer than you should?

If this sounds like you, you're probably getting overwhelmed too easily. Giving up on or avoiding chores altogether usually results in getting further and further behind. Knowing that chores are stacking up can worsen your depression, especially if it makes you feel bad about yourself. Here's how it works:

- When you get overwhelmed, you're often telling yourself, "I can't handle it," and you feel extremely tense. When you walk away from a task, you're telling yourself, "You'll be OK now that you got away from it," and you feel more relaxed.
- You are accidentally teaching yourself that doing tough tasks is stressful or bad and walking away from them makes you feel better. This means that the next time you are faced with a difficult problem, you are more likely to walk away than to handle it.
- In the process you begin to lose your self-confidence.
- When your confidence is low, you are less likely to make yourself deal with stressful situations.
- In the meantime, problems or tasks can get bigger and harder to handle.
- All of this makes you feel more depressed.

The best way to handle this situation is to break it down and take it on!

How to Break It Down and Take It On!

The way to cope with the feeling of being overwhelmed and still make some progress toward your goals is to change the way you look at a task or problem. Whether you're talking about cleaning a house you've neglected for months, catching up on your income tax filing, or getting a job, you can turn a big overwhelming task into smaller, more manageable parts. It's all in how you look at it.

If you see a messy apartment as a disaster area that will take weeks to clean, it can seem too overwhelming to take on. If you want to go to work, but think about all the little things that must be done to prepare yourself to work, to find available positions, and to convince someone to hire you, the sheer magnitude of the task can stop you in your tracks. When you're depressed, if your motivation is low, you can't imagine how to begin. If your concentration is poor, you may not be able to keep your mind focused long enough to get organized. If your energy is low, you may be too tired to do the work. All of this taken together contributes to your feeling completely overwhelmed.

Depression + A big task to do = Feeling overwhelmed

If solving a big problem would make you feel better, then try the steps in the next section to break it down into smaller and more manageable parts and take it on one step at a time.

How to Break It Down

- **Step 1: Don't tell yourself that it has to be done all at once.** You might prefer to take care of the whole thing in one day, but this may not be reasonable. Write out some reminders to yourself on Worksheet 5.11 that might help you set realistic goals for getting things done.
- Amanda is a bit of a perfectionist and expects herself to be on top of things at all times. When she has tried to tell herself that it was OK to do a small amount of work at a time, it didn't work because another part of her responded by saying that she *should* be able to get it all done. In fact, she used to be able to do big chores in one day when she wasn't so depressed. If you are like Amanda, you may have to work at cutting yourself some slack. It's better to do a small amount of work at a time than to do nothing at all. Something is better than nothing. Try saying that to yourself when your perfectionism sets too high a standard.

| worksheet 5.11 | **One Thing at a Time** |

Things I can say to myself about doing one thing at a time:
(e.g., *Even if I can't do it all, doing something is better than doing nothing.*)

From *The Bipolar Workbook* by Monica Ramirez Basco. Copyright 2006 by The Guilford Press. Permission to photocopy this form is granted to purchasers of this book for personal use only (see copyright page for details).

- **Step 2: Write down all the steps involved** in solving your problem or completing your task. You may not like writing things down, but taking it out of your head and putting it on paper will help you feel less overwhelmed. Try writing down your ideas on Worksheet 5.12 and see if it works for you.

Paul found it helpful to write out a list of steps it would take to get caught up with a research paper he needed to write for class. When he broke it down, it seemed more manageable to him.

Amanda, on the other hand, started to write down the steps it would take to clean her house and got overwhelmed with the number of things she had to do. She put down the list and just started cleaning the house. It worked better for her to go on to Step 3.

- **Step 3: Pick a place to start.** There may be an obvious first step, but in most cases doing anything, even if it is out of sequence, is better than doing nothing. If you feel the urge to do more than one step, try to resist it. If you take on too much, you will feel overwhelmed all over again. Pick your first step and write it down on Worksheet 5.13. Seeing it in writing can help you keep your commitment to yourself.

Raquel would get behind on paying bills from time to time. She hated the task because it always reminded her that they had very little money. Because she often avoided paying bills, she did not have an organized system for keeping the bills together, knowing where her checkbook was, or knowing the due dates of each. She thought about trying to create a system, but that would take more time than she wanted to give to the task. Instead, she found her checkbook and paid bills off and on throughout the day as she found them. Raquel knew it was not the most efficient way to go about it, but at least it got done.

---

worksheet 5.12 | **Steps to Accomplish**

The steps I want to accomplish:

| worksheet 5.13 | **The First Step** |

This is where I am going to start:

How to Take It On

- **Step 1: Pick a day and time to start.** Make an appointment with yourself to begin the first step of your chore. Choose a time that is realistic, when lots of interruptions are unlikely to occur and your other obligations are unlikely to interfere. Schedule it for when you are likely to have time and energy.

- **Step 2: Do the first step** even if you're not in the mood, not feeling motivated, or can think of a dozen other things you would rather do. Tell yourself that making a little bit of progress is better than making no progress at all.

Many people complain about being unmotivated and uninterested in taking care of unpleasant tasks, especially when just thinking about it makes them feel overwhelmed. They put things off until they feel motivated to act, but that feeling rarely comes. There is no real magic to increasing your motivation or making yourself take action. When it comes down to it, it's just a matter of deciding that it's in your best interest to take action. You take the first step despite all of your resistance and excuses because you believe it's the right thing to do. For that moment, you ignore the negative emotions that paralyze you and just get started. Once you see yourself act, your motivation will begin to return.

- **Step 3: Cross each step off the list as it is completed.** Give yourself a pat on the back or treat yourself to something fun or pleasurable for taking some action. Avoid telling yourself that it doesn't matter because you have so much more to do. You have to make the work worthwhile. If you are someone who is motivated by the relief you feel when something gets done, completing the task may be the only reward you need. If the task you are trying to do is difficult for you and does not give you a lot of pleasure, you will have to find another way to give yourself positive reinforcement for getting it done. This is an important step because it gives you a reason to go on with the next part of the task. Think of a possible reward to give to yourself. It does not have to be a Disneyland-size reward. Allowing yourself a rest, eating an ice cream cone, watching a favorite TV show, or taking a bubble bath can be rewarding. Plan ahead for your reward and write it down on Worksheet 5.14 to help you remember to do it.

- Raquel's reward for getting the bills paid was having a cup of tea and polishing her nails.
- Amanda's reward for taking action toward her goals is getting a break from self-criticism for her procrastination.
- Paul's reward for finishing the term paper will be eating his favorite dessert after dinner.

- **Step 4: Select the next part** of the task to do and schedule a time to do it. Repeat steps 1 through 4 until you are done. When you have completed your task, give yourself some credit or a reward, or brag to someone who will understand what you've accomplished!

Disqualifying the Accomplishment

Raquel expects a great deal from herself even when she is feeling depressed. She doesn't cut herself any slack for having low energy at times or difficulty concentrating. She uses the step-by-step method described when she gets overwhelmed and stuck, but when she accomplishes each piece, instead of giving herself praise, she

---

worksheet 5.14 | **Possible Rewards**

When I am able to take action, I will give myself the following reward:

From *The Bipolar Workbook* by Monica Ramirez Basco. Copyright 2006 by The Guilford Press. Permission to photocopy this form is granted to purchasers of this book for personal use only (see copyright page for details).

criticizes herself for not having finished the task sooner or not having done a better job.

Beating yourself up for accomplishing tasks is not a way to get motivated. If you were coaching someone else—for example, a child or a student—you would not berate the person for not completing the tasks sooner or better. If you did, the child or student would stop performing for you. You are no different.

People with bipolar disorder who also have a perfectionistic streak can do themselves harm by withholding encouragement and praise until a high standard of performance is met. When you struggle with mood swings and all the other symptoms of bipolar disorder, perfection is hard to come by. If this sounds like you, try not to defeat yourself by expecting more than is reasonable. Sometimes you have to pat yourself on the back just for getting up in the morning because sometimes getting yourself out of bed *is* a major accomplishment.

The Lethargy Cycle

It's easy to get caught in a lethargy cycle when you're feeling depressed. Depression usually causes you to have low energy, to get fatigued easily, and to lose interest in your usual activities. When you do less, you feel worse. This feeds your depression.

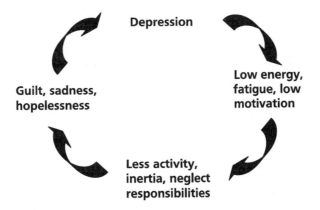

To overcome lethargy, you have to find a way to break the cycle. In the following sections two methods are described for breaking the lethargy cycle by finding a way to take action. Like the last exercise, both have to do with simplifying what you have to do so that it does not feel so overwhelming and taking one step at a time.

If you've been stuck in a lethargy cycle for some time, you might find it particularly hard to find your way out. You will probably take action only if you have a really good reason to do so. Therefore, before you work your way through the following exercises, take a minute and think of reasons it would be good for you to break your lethargy cycle and take action. Write down your reasons to take action on Worksheet 5.15. Amanda's reasons are that she has to take care of her children, she is tired of being in a funk, and she feels better about herself when she does something other than lie on the couch. Paul's reasons for getting out of a slump of inactivity are that he has a lot to do, things will only get worse the longer he neglects them, and he hates being different from everyone else. Raquel rarely gets into slumps anymore since she has learned to control her symptoms, but when she has been lethargic in the past she wanted out of it because even though she was not taking action she could not stop thinking about how she should get up and get something done. She may have looked like she was resting, but her guilt and self-criticism made it anything but restful.

Activity Scheduling

Some people find it helpful to get themselves on a schedule when depressed, inactive, or disorganized. If you don't have a regular schedule of activities, such as work or school, it's easy to waste a lot of time doing nothing at all. The problem with doing nothing is that you might be missing out on things that would make you feel better about yourself or give you a sense of accomplishment. You also might be missing out on opportunities to have fun. Engaging in enjoyable activities can lift your mood. When that happens, you will often feel more energetic and motivated to take care of other aspects of your life.

Worksheet 5.16 comes in two parts: an Activity Schedule for Sunday through Tuesday and one for Wednesday through Saturday. You can make a schedule for the

---

| worksheet 5.15 | **Reasons to Take Action** |

My reasons for taking action

_____

_____

_____

_____

_____

whole week or make plans one day at a time. To make the best use of Activity Schedules, make time the night before to plan for the following day. When you know what you'll be doing tomorrow, you avoid wasting time and prevent your low motivation from taking complete control. Some tips for completing your activity schedule are listed in the table below.

Tips for Completing Your Activity Schedule

- Fill in the time you plan to wake up and go to bed each day.
- Write in regularly scheduled activities like work or appointments.
- Plan at least one small pleasurable activity each day.
- Schedule time to accomplish one task each day.
- Be realistic with your planning. Don't schedule too much.

"A" List and "B" List

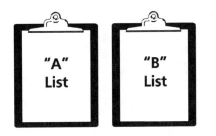

A simpler method for planning than activity scheduling is to make a short list each day of things you absolutely have to do and things you would like to do if you had the time and energy. The things you have to do will become your "A" list. You should never have more than a few items on that list for any day. "A" list items are things that cannot wait, such as paying a bill, getting food from the store, or attending an appointment.

The items on your "B" list will include things you would like to do if you had the time. They do not absolutely have to be done that day, but if time and energy permit, you would really like to do them. This might include running an errand ahead of time rather than waiting until it's urgent or refilling a prescription before you take the last pill. "B" list items can also be fun activities like visiting a friend, working on a hobby, or reading a book for enjoyment. There should never be more than a few items on your "B" list for any one day, especially if your "A" list is likely to take a lot of time.

The goal is to try to finish your "A" list activities before your begin your "B" list activities. Like the goal-setting exercise you may have done, this will allow you to do the most important things first, solve problems, and have a sense of accomplishment. Any leftover items can be carried on to the next day.

Here is an example of the "A" and "B" lists Paul made after completing the Goal-Setting Worksheet.

Activity Schedule, Sunday–Tuesday

Put an × in the box after completing each task.

Time	Date: _____ Sunday	Monday	Tuesday
9:00 A.M.	❏	❏	❏
10:00	❏	❏	❏
11:00	❏	❏	❏
12:00 P.M.	❏	❏	❏
1:00	❏	❏	❏
2:00	❏	❏	❏
3:00	❏	❏	❏
4:00	❏	❏	❏
5:00	❏	❏	❏
6:00	❏	❏	❏
7:00	❏	❏	❏
8:00	❏	❏	❏
9:00	❏	❏	❏

Activity Schedule, Wednesday–Saturday

Put an × in the box after completing each task.

Time	Date: _____ Wednesday	Thursday	Friday	Saturday
9:00 A.M.	❑	❑	❑	❑
10:00	❑	❑	❑	❑
11:00	❑	❑	❑	❑
12:00 P.M.	❑	❑	❑	❑
1:00	❑	❑	❑	❑
2:00	❑	❑	❑	❑
3:00	❑	❑	❑	❑
4:00	❑	❑	❑	❑
5:00	❑	❑	❑	❑
6:00	❑	❑	❑	❑
7:00	❑	❑	❑	❑
8:00	❑	❑	❑	❑
9:00	❑	❑	❑	❑

My "A" List

Things I need to do today

1. Pay the rent.
2. Get Alice's phone number from her friend.
3. Ask Alice out for Friday night.

My "B" List

Things I'd like to do when I finish my "A" list

1. Wash one load of laundry—underwear.
2. Call the windshield repair company to schedule a repair on my car.
3. Work on the research paper due in class next week.

The Desire for Change

It is normal to want change in your life from time to time. We all get the urge to change our hairstyle, move to a new place, repaint our house, rearrange our furniture, learn a new hobby, change jobs, or otherwise make our lives more interesting. There is nothing wrong with change. It can become a negative, however, if too many changes are attempted at the same time—for example, when many projects get started but few are finished. Hypomania and mania tend to drive the urge for change and can make people take action without fully thinking things through. If you're easily distracted, you could start on making a change at home, like rearranging your furniture, but have something else catch your eye, like working on photo albums or cleaning out a closet. Before the second task can be finished, a third might come to mind, especially if you're at the stage in hypomania where you have a lot of creative ideas. If you could handle all the changes you started, it would not likely be a problem. Unfortunately, as you get distracted or when you have too many ideas, you can become disorganized and eventually overwhelmed with all that needs to be done. If depression follows a hypomanic or manic period, these unfinished projects or chores, disarray in your environment, or excessive money spent on materials needed to make the changes you wanted can make you feel even worse.

There are a few strategies for coping with the urge to change. One is to put some time between having an idea for change and taking action on it. During that pause you have time to ask yourself a few questions, such as:

- *Do I really want to make this change?*
- *Is it worth my time and energy?*

- *How much effort am I willing to put out?*
- *Does anyone else think this is a good idea?*
- *Am I having a general urge for change, or am I really dissatisfied with how things are?*

If you believe the desire for change is driven by hypomania or mania, another strategy is to take the necessary precautions to control symptoms and then ask yourself if there is something small you can change to satisfy the need. Instead of buying a new car, can you wash and wax the one you have? Instead of moving to a new apartment, is there something you can change in your old one that will make it more attractive or better organized? Can you rearrange things to make more space rather than getting a bigger place? If you have the urge to change your hair color, pick a temporary coloring product that will wash out if you change your mind. Rather than getting an extreme haircut, try styling it differently or ask a friend or hair specialist to do it for you. If you want a new look, work with the clothes you have rather than buying new things. If you need accessories, go to a discount or re-sale store before spending money you might later regret. If you want to make bigger changes such as in boyfriends, girlfriends, lovers, or spouses, read Chapter 9 first. In that chapter you will learn how to slow down, focus your attention, and make good decisions.

What's Next?

This chapter was full of information on things you can do to prevent symptoms from returning or prevent them from worsening once they start. These strategies will serve you best if you can put them to use in your day-to-day life. There is a lot to remember to do, so you may have to reread this chapter when you think your symptoms are returning and follow the instructions that apply to your situation at that time. To make it easier on yourself, you may want to choose one area to work on at a time, such as regulating your sleep or keeping yourself from getting over-stimulated.

One of the best precautions you can take in controlling bipolar disorder is to be consistent in taking medications. This is a touchy subject for many people. That is why the next chapter is dedicated fully to the issue of taking medications. Whether you have decided not to take medications at all or are perfectly consistent in taking them, you will probably find Chapter 6 thought provoking.

chapter six

Getting the Most Out
of Medication

In this chapter you will:

✓ Evaluate your beliefs about taking medication for bipolar disorder.
✓ Figure out what keeps you from taking medication regularly.
✓ Use behavioral contracts to create a personal plan for treatment.
✓ Learn what you should do if you want to take a break from medications.

If you've been diagnosed with bipolar disorder, more than likely you have been prescribed medication to control your symptoms. Taking medications for this illness is not like taking medications for a cold or an infection or to control pain. Following are some basic facts about the medication treatment of bipolar disorder.

• **Fact 1: Medication is required to fully control the symptoms of this disorder and to prevent symptoms from returning once they have remitted.** A significant amount of research has been conducted on the treatment of depression and mania in bipolar disorder, and the results consistently show that people tend to do better with medication than without it. Mark how strongly you believe this on Worksheet 6.1.

• **Fact 2: Most people who have bipolar disorder do not like taking medication. And most go through periods of time when they stop it altogether, take it less consistently, or alter the regimen on their own to try to make it more tolerable.** The research on adherence with treatment for bipolar disorder shows that the majority of people with bipolar disorder take some of their medications most of the time and all of their medications some of the time. A smaller group of people take all their medications all of the time, particularly those who are organized and consistent about other things in their lives. And there are some people who stop taking all of

| worksheet 6.1 | **Belief in Fact 1** |

How strongly do you believe Fact 1?

0%	50%	100%
I do not believe this at all	I'm not sure yet	I know this to be true

If you don't strongly believe it, what would it take to convince you?

How could you get the information you needed to explore this idea?

---

their medications altogether. Over your lifetime of dealing with bipolar disorder there is a good chance that you will have times when you take less medication than your doctor would prefer or take it less consistently than prescribed. Look over Worksheet 6.2 and mark the answers that apply to you.

• **Fact 3: Most medications prescribed for the symptoms of bipolar disorder do not work unless they are taken very consistently and at a dose high enough to have a positive effect.** This may sound obvious, but because the mood swings come and go, it's easy to assume that medication can be used off and on.

Tommy challenged his doctor when he insisted that Tommy keep taking Depakote and lithium even after his mania subsided.

> *I don't see why I have to. I had strep throat last year that got really bad. I had to be on two different antibiotics to finally kill it. But when the infection was gone, I didn't need to keep taking more antibiotics just to keep from ever getting another one. So why should I keep taking lithium? It makes me tired. I can hardly concentrate in class, and I'm not manic anymore.*

Tommy made an interesting point that on the surface does not sound illogical. Tommy's doctor explained that bipolar disorder is not an infection or virus that

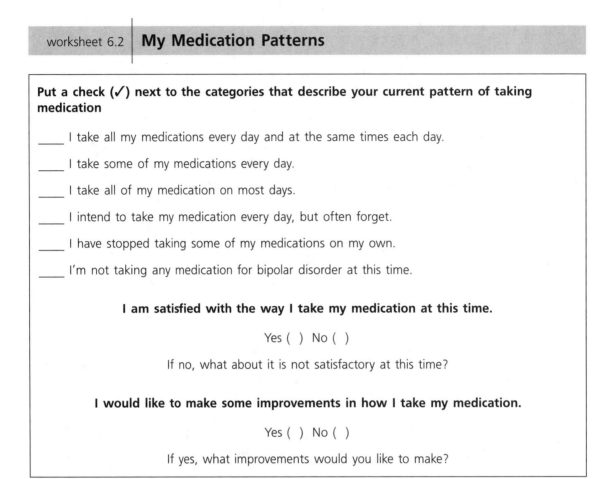

worksheet 6.2 | **My Medication Patterns**

Put a check (✓) next to the categories that describe your current pattern of taking medication

____ I take all my medications every day and at the same times each day.

____ I take some of my medications every day.

____ I take all of my medication on most days.

____ I intend to take my medication every day, but often forget.

____ I have stopped taking some of my medications on my own.

____ I'm not taking any medication for bipolar disorder at this time.

I am satisfied with the way I take my medication at this time.

Yes ( ) No ( )

If no, what about it is not satisfactory at this time?

I would like to make some improvements in how I take my medication.

Yes ( ) No ( )

If yes, what improvements would you like to make?

goes away. The medications control the symptoms and can help to keep mania and depression from returning, but they do not fix the underlying biological problem that produces the symptoms. It's similar to having diabetes in this way. People take medication to control the symptoms of diabetes, but so far there is no real cure.

Tommy has been told this before and seems to understand the concept but is not ready to fully accept the idea that he has a chronic mental illness. He went along with treatment while he was feeling bad, but he never envisioned having to take medication for the rest of his life.

Would you agree with Tommy? He doesn't buy the idea that he might have to take medication continuously for the rest of his life. Take a minute to think this over and respond to the questions in Worksheet 6.3.

• **Fact 4: Taking medication daily for bipolar disorder is not just about the pills; it is about accepting a fate you may not be ready to take on.** Amanda still struggles with this idea. The intellectual side of her understands that she has an illness that requires treatment. She is tired of struggling against the illness and against the doctors and really wants to have more stability in her life. The emotional side of her, however, finds it unacceptable. She is angry that she got this illness and none of her sisters got it. She is angry with her mother for passing on her "bad" genes. She is frustrated with psychiatrists because they can't find a cure. At a recent support group meeting, Amanda had this to say:

It's not fair. It shouldn't have to be this way. It's not right. Why should I have to be the one that deals with this? Why should I have to take multiple medications when other people have to take only one? Why can't they find a cure? I hate taking medicines. I don't even like taking aspirins. I'm a nurse. I'm supposed to help others, not be a patient myself. This was not the way it was supposed to turn out!

Raquel was at the same meeting and had this to offer Amanda:

You're right that it's not fair. It's never fair that some people have to suffer more than others. And it's frustrating that scientists seem to be getting closer to a

---

| worksheet 6.3 | **Belief in Fact 3** |

How strongly do you believe Fact 3?

0%	50%	100%
I do not believe this at all	I'm not sure yet	I know this to be true

If you do not strongly believe it, what do you think would be a more accurate statement about taking medication?

What would it take to change your mind?

---

cure for so many other diseases but can't get a handle on this one. I agree that it should not be this way. You have a right to be mad. But then what do you do? I stayed mad for many years after I was diagnosed with bipolar disorder. I was even angrier when my little granddaughter was diagnosed with it. I blamed the doctors, God, and myself. I cried about it, prayed for it to go away or to be a mistake, and even tried to pretend it wasn't real. But for all my complaining and anger and tears, the spells of depression kept coming back. Staying angry didn't get me very far. Fixing the problem as best I could by following my doctor's orders gave me a chance at a new life. You have to get the big picture, Amanda. Ask yourself what you're going to do once you finish crying or being angry. Ask yourself what you can do to make tomorrow better.

Give some thought to what Amanda and Raquel had to say and make some notes about your ideas on Worksheet 6.4.

• **Fact 5: Most people are not open-minded about mental illnesses or accepting of those who have one.** Amanda is a nurse, but she tells her friends that she would rather have diabetes than bipolar disorder. She would still have to take medication for the rest of her life and modify her lifestyle, but at least she wouldn't be considered "crazy." Society is slowly changing and beginning to understand that mental illnesses are illnesses like those in any other organ of the body. However, we have not evolved in our sophistication enough to fully accept people who are mentally ill. Having a mental illness may not make you any more open-minded. Even people who have bipolar disorder can be biased against other people who have mental ill-

---

| worksheet 6.4 | **View of Having Bipolar Disorder** |

What are your thoughts about Amanda's attitude?

What is your opinion about Raquel's advice?

---

nesses. If you think that having a mental illness is unacceptable or is a character flaw, or that mental illnesses are not real illnesses, you will have a hard time accepting the disorder within yourself. If you can't accept that it exists, you will find it a challenge to go along with its treatment. Give this some thought before you respond to the questions on Worksheet 6.5.

• **Fact 6: Most medications do not work for everyone. It is not always possible to know ahead of time whether or not a medication will work for you,** and few people find the right combination of medications on the first try. These facts can make it very hard for you to keep trying out different medications until your doctor finds one that works, because while you are trying out different ones you continue to experience the discomfort of symptoms. Medication changes can also be expensive, and not all health plans cover the medications your doctor might want you to try. It takes tremendous patience on your part to stick with this trial-and-error approach. In the long run it's usually worth it, but it's normal to have doubts along the way. Make some notes on Worksheet 6.6 on how you've coped so far with medication changes.

• **Fact 7: If you discontinue taking medications for bipolar disorder, you're at a high risk of relapsing and suffering through the consequences of becoming severely depressed or severely manic.** The common cause of relapse in bipolar disorder is going off medication. Sometimes symptoms return immediately, but other times there may be a delay. It's the delays that will give you the impression that you don't really need medication. If you are unsure about whether this applies to you, go back and

---

| worksheet 6.5 | **Your Opinion of Mental Illness** |

When you see people with mental illnesses in your doctor's office or other places, what do you think about them?

Does that view apply to you too?

| worksheet 6.6 | **Thoughts on How to Stick with Treatment** |

If you are someone who has been through numerous medications before finding one that worked, how did you keep yourself going through that frustrating process?

If you get into that situation again, what would you like to be able to remind yourself about the value of sticking with treatment even if medicines have to be changed or added?

If you are currently in the process of trying to find the right medication, what are your reasons for hanging in there? What advice might you give to others?

review the Life Chart you created in Chapter 3. Look closely for a link between times that medications were discontinued and times when symptoms returned.

• **Fact 8: If you discontinue taking medications for bipolar disorder and then try to start them up again when your symptoms return, they may not be as effective.** The life-charting research mentioned in Chapter 3 showed that when mood-stabilizing medications such as lithium were discontinued and then resumed at a later date, they were found to be less effective or were completely ineffective in controlling symptoms. Many have found this to be the case for antidepressant medications as well.

When Paul was a teenager, he tried to make the following argument with his doctor and his parents.

If episodes of depression and mania occur only from time to time with periods of normal mood in between, isn't it possible that during those in-between times

I don't need medication? If I went five years without another mania, those would be five years I could have been off medication.

Paul would not be wrong in theory, but since recurrences of depression and mania are not always predictable and usually do not follow a uniform pattern, it's not possible to know when the next episode is coming. What is known is that without consistent medication treatment, as a person ages the time between episodes of depression and mania will get shorter and each episode itself will tend to get longer. It took a few more experiences with severe depression before Paul was willing to concede this point.

• **Fact 9: Even if you have come to terms with having bipolar disorder and agree to take medication regularly, a number of things can keep you from following the treatment regimen as prescribed by your doctor.**

Sometimes there are **practical reasons**, like:

- *I ran out of medicines.*
- *I forgot to take them.*
- *I don't have any money to buy my medicines.*
- *I don't have a ride to the pharmacy to pick up my medicines.*

Sometimes there are **family reasons**, like:

- *My mom worries about my taking medicines.*
- *My brother had a reaction to these medicines, so I'm afraid to take them.*
- *My family doesn't understand why I have to take medicines.*

Sometimes the reason that people don't take their medications regularly is the **medication itself**, like:

- *It makes me sleepy all day.*
- *It makes me gain weight.*
- *There are too many of them.*

Sometimes people have **personal reasons** for not wanting to take medications at all, like:

- *I don't like having to depend on medicines.*
- *I'm afraid I'm going to get hooked on them.*
- *I'm feeling fine. I don't need them anymore.*
- *They don't really help me.*

Sometimes the reason for not taking medicine as prescribed has something to do with **the doctor or the clinic**, like:

- *The doctor doesn't seem to really understand me.*
- *The doctor rushed through my appointment and didn't take time to listen to me.*

- *I don't like my doctor, the nurse, or the clinic.*
- *I disagree with the doctor's ideas.*

The sections that follow describe a number of strategies for helping you be as consistent with your medication as you can, as often as possible. Chapter 7 will help you work through your hesitations about accepting the diagnosis of bipolar disorder so that this obstacle will no longer stand in the way of your medication treatment.

Planning Ahead with Behavioral Contracts

A behavioral contract is a structure for setting treatment goals, anticipating things that could interfere with your progress, and eliminating them or learning to cope with them when they occur. Goals to address in the behavioral contract might include doing what you can to take medication regularly and as it is prescribed as well as mustering the self-discipline to use the exercises in this book or to follow the advice of your therapist or counselor. When you make a contract with yourself, you are committing to a plan that will help you gain better control over your illness.

The behavioral contract presented in Worksheet 6.8 has **three parts**. In the **first part**, you state your treatment plans. This will include your plan for taking medication, using the methods in this book, and participating in any other types of treatment you have decided to begin. Those might include individual or group psychotherapy, or support group meetings such as those offered by Alcoholics Anonymous (*www.AA.org*) or the Depression and Bipolar Support Alliance (*www. DBSAlliance.org*).

In the **second part** of the behavioral contract you make a list of things that could keep you from accomplishing your goals, like the ones listed under Fact 9. This will help you plan ahead for times when you might stray from your treatment goals.

If you know what can interfere with your goals, you can make a plan to avoid

worksheet 6.7 | **Obstacles to Adherence**

Go back through the list on pages 125–126 and **put a check** next to the reasons you have ever had for not adhering to your medication regimen as prescribed over the time you've been treated for bipolar disorder. **Circle the challenges you still encounter** when trying to take your medication as consistently as possible.

such obstacles or to cope with them once they occur. In the **third part** of the behavioral contract you will be making a plan to deal with each of the obstacles to treatment that you identified in the second part.

Part I: Your Goals

In Part I of your personal plan for treatment, write in the medications you plan to take on a regular basis. Be specific about the dose and the times of day you want to take them.

In addition to taking medications, you probably have personal goals you would like to accomplish as part of your therapy or self-help plan. Your goals might include getting yourself to stop a behavior, change a behavior, or learn something new. Sometimes your personal goals include coping better with other people. Try to be as specific as possible. For example, don't set a goal such as "being a better person." That is too general. Instead, think of a way in which you would like to change yourself. Maybe you want to stop procrastinating, get a job, control your anger, or communicate more assertively with others. These would be reasonable treatment goals.

Part II: The Obstacles

Think back to times in the past when you might have skipped medications intentionally, accidentally missed a few, run out, or decided to quit even when your doctor thought that was a bad idea. In Part II of your treatment plan, write in the factors that might have kept you from sticking with the treatment plan. Review the list of obstacles presented under Fact 9 and write any that apply to you in Part II of the behavioral contract. Following are some questions to help you recall the factors that might have kept you from taking medications in the past as you had intended or as your doctor had recommended. Add any pertinent factors to Part II.

- What kinds of things might have influenced your decision to discontinue medication?
- Did your mood or your state of mind have anything to do with it? If so, what kind of mood or symptoms could make you want to skip doses or stop altogether?
- Did anyone else encourage you to quit taking medicines?
- Do you have any personal qualities or weaknesses that could have made you less consistent with treatment? How about forgetfulness, lack of organization, or impatience?
- Were you overly confident that you could handle things without medication?
- Did you have a negative attitude or just get tired of taking medication?

MY BEHAVIORAL CONTRACT

Part I: My Goals

I intend to follow this plan for taking medication as often as possible:

Type of medication	Dose	When I'll take it
_____	_____	_____
_____	_____	_____
_____	_____	_____
_____	_____	_____
_____	_____	_____

My other goals for treatment are as follows:

Therapy:

_____

_____

_____

Self-help plan:

_____

_____

_____

Part II: The Obstacles

It is possible that the following factors could keep me from taking medication regularly:

_____	_____
_____	_____
_____	_____
_____	_____

It is possible that the following factors could keep me from participating in therapy or from using other self-help methods:

_____   _____

_____   _____

_____   _____

_____   _____

Part III: The Plan

The following is my plan for overcoming the obstacles I listed in Part II.

Issue   Plan

_____   _____

_____   _____

_____   _____

_____   _____

_____   _____

_____   _____

_____   _____

_____   _____

_____   _____

_____   _____

_____   _____

_____   _____

_____   _____

_____   _____

_____   _____

_____   _____

Part III: The Plan

Now that you know the possible pitfalls, it's time to make a plan for how you will handle each if it occurs. If you make a plan now, you will be better prepared to head off problems with medication before they interfere with your progress and recovery.

The sections that follow offer some suggestions for common problems with taking medications regularly. Pick the solutions that suit you best or modify these suggestions to fit your own situation. Write your ideas for coping with these situations in Part III of your behavioral contract.

"I sometimes forget to take my medication. What should I do?"

Suggestion 1

Always take your medicine at the same time each day. Make it a routine, just like putting on your shoes each day or brushing your teeth.

Suggestion 2

Use a divided pillbox for your medication. Check the box midday to be sure you've taken your medication. Put the box in a place you are likely to see each day. If you see it, you'll be more likely to take your medicine.

Suggestion 3

Write a note to yourself that reminds you to take your medication. Put the note in a place that you will see each day. Some common places to put reminder notes include your refrigerator, near your bathroom mirror, or in your car.

Suggestion 4

Most people have a daily routine or set of daily habits. Some examples of daily routine or habits include:

- Getting up at the same time each day.
- Brushing their teeth in the morning.
- Drinking their morning coffee.
- Getting dressed for the day.
- Watching certain TV shows.

A way to remember to take your medications regularly is to take them at the same time that you complete one of your other daily routines or habits. For example, you might take your medicine with your morning coffee.

"I don't think I need these medicines anymore. What should I do?"

Suggestion 1

Before you decide to stop taking your medication, talk with your doctor about your concerns. Some medications should be taken daily even when you're feeling better. The purpose of these medications is to keep your symptoms from returning. If you're feeling fine now, it's probably because the medication is working well.

Suggestion 2

The urge to stop taking medication and feeling like you don't need it anymore might really be a sign that the illness is getting worse. To be certain, before stopping any medications, talk with your doctor. Be sure you are making a good decision. The desire to stop taking medication is sometimes a signal that the symptoms are returning or are getting worse.

If you are depressed, it can feel as if the medication is not helping, that nothing can help. Sometimes people feel hopeless or overwhelmed and don't know what to do. They may end up thinking it would be better to stop taking their medication.

This way of thinking is actually a sign that depression is getting worse. It would not be the best time to stop taking medication, but it would be a good time to see your doctor and ask for help.

If you are getting manic, you might feel really good, better than usual, and think you don't need medication anymore. This is called *hypomania*. It is the early stage of mania. Hypomania can very quickly turn into mania, especially if you stop taking your medications. Before you make the decision to stop your medicines, ask someone else for an opinion on how you are doing,

"Some of my family members don't think I should take medication. What should I do?"

When family members discourage you from taking medications, it's usually because they have worries or concerns about them. Sometimes people hear stories about medications that have scared them. In trying to protect you from harm, they might tell you not to take them or question your need for them.

The usual problem is that family members may not understand your illness or the purpose of taking medications. They might need more information or education from your doctor or therapist.

Here are some ways to get them the information they need.

Suggestion 1

Ask one of your family members to come with you to your next doctor's appointment. If only one family member can come to your appointment, choose one who can talk with the other members of your family and share what is learned during the visit.

Tell your doctor that the family is worried about your taking medications. The doctor will help your family understand more about your illness and will explain the purpose of the medications. Your family members will have an opportunity to ask questions about their concerns or fears.

Suggestion 2

Ask your doctor for some written information about your illness and its treatment. Give this information to your family members.

Suggestion 3

Invite your family members to go with you to a support group meeting such as one held by the Depression and Bipolar Support Alliance (DBSA) or the National Alliance of the Mentally Ill (NAMI). These groups provide information for family members about mental illnesses and their treatments.

Suggestion 4

Thank your family members for their concern. Tell them where they can get more information about your treatment. Let them know that you have decided to take the medication to control your symptoms.

"I don't like the way my medication makes me feel."

Side effects are one of the most common reasons that people stop taking their medications. For many medications, however, the side effects are temporary. They occur when you first begin taking medication or when you change your dose. If you miss taking your medication for a few days and start up again, your side effects may return. Sometimes side effects from medication can persist even after you've been taking medication for some time.

Suggestion 1

Talk to your doctor about the way your medications make you feel. Ask if the discomforts are a result of medication or a separate problem altogether. If you're experiencing side effects, ask your doctor how long they are likely to last and whether anything can be done about it. Follow the doctor's advice. If you give it enough time and still feel uncomfortable, talk with your doctor again.

Suggestion 2

Because doctors are more familiar with the side effects of medication than you, they may not be as concerned as you when they occur. They may assess your problem and tell you that the symptoms will pass. If you sense a lack of concern or that he or she too quickly dismissed your complaints, calmly tell the doctor what you are thinking. Ask why he or she does not seem worried. Make sure you've made it clear just how bothersome the side effects are.

Suggestion 3

If the side effects are not likely to go away, consider whether the benefits you get from the medication may be worth tolerating the side effects. If the medication keeps you from getting depressed or manic, maybe it's worth tolerating the annoying side effects. When you're feeling well, it's easy to focus on the side effect as being the biggest annoyance in your life. When you were having severe symptoms, you felt so bad that the side effects may not have mattered. Think it through before you stop your medication.

"I'm afraid to take medications."

It's normal to feel afraid of new treatments. You may wonder if you've received the right diagnosis and whether the medications you were prescribed are really the best choices for you. If you've heard stories about bad experiences that people have had when taking medication, you might be concerned that you could have a bad experience also.

Suggestion 1

Ask your doctor plenty of questions about the medicine. Start by asking some of the following:

- *Why did you choose these particular medications for me?*
- *Could there be any bad side effects? If so, what are they?*
- *What should I do if I start to feel the side effects?*
- *Whom should I call? Should I stop them right away?*

Suggestion 2

Talk to other people who have taken the same medication and have done all right. Ask them about the things that worry you.

If any of the situations previously described apply to you, you might be able to add some of the suggestions for coping to Part III of your behavioral contract. To help you get started, Amanda's completed behavioral contract is provided as an example. Amanda has had difficulty being consistent with her medications for many years. She wants to have a more stable life and is eager to do her part to make that happen. She has struggled with acceptance of the illness but feels that she has turned the corner and is ready to deal with it.

After you've created your behavioral contract, give a copy to your doctor and your therapist. Put a copy for yourself in a place where you will see it from time to time. Make it your mission to review the plan periodically.

If new situations occur that make you think about stopping your medications or at least skipping a few doses, add them to you plan, talk them over with your doctor or therapist, and try to figure out a way to keep them from interfering with your goals.

Find a time to regularly review your goals. Amanda has decided that she will review the plan before each appointment with her psychiatrist. Raquel has been on the same medication regimen for years and has no trouble sticking with it. She reviews her plan when she sees her doctor every 6 months. Paul has his plan on his computer as a screen saver. It pops up from time to time to remind him of his goals. He updates it regularly. Tommy is not quite ready to make a behavioral contract. He needs time to work on his acceptance of the illness before he is willing to make a long-term commitment to treatment. He is going to read ahead to Chapter 7 and come back to the contract idea at a later date.

What You Should Do If You Really Want to Take a Break from Medication Treatment

- Talk it over with your doctor. Discuss the pros and cons of doing so.
- Be certain that decreasing medications is a reasonable idea and not a manic idea. If you're uncertain, review the Mood Symptoms Worksheet that you created in Chapter 4 to determine whether you're having any symptoms of mania or depression. If so, postpone your plan until your symptoms are more stable and reevaluate.

Amanda's Worksheet 6.8

Part I: My Goals

I intend to follow this plan for taking medication as often as possible:

Type of medication	Dose	When I'll take it
Lithium	900 mg	at night

My other goals for treatment are as follows:

Therapy:

Meet with my therapist regularly for at least 6 months and work through this
workbook together.

Self-help plan:

I will go to AA meetings at least twice each week even when I don't think I need
it. I will also go to support group meetings every other month. I will make time
each week to work on the exercises in this workbook.

Part II: The Obstacles

It is possible that the following factors could keep me from taking medication regularly:

Losing patience with a slow recovery	Getting annoyed with the doctor
Weight gain	

Amanda's Worksheet 6.8 *(cont.)*

It is possible that the following factors could keep me from participating in therapy or from using other self-help methods:

Being too busy to attend group

meetings

Not having a quiet moment at home to

work on the exercises in this book

Part III: The Plan

The following is my plan for overcoming the obstacles I listed in Part II.

Issue

Plan

Impatience:

Remember that progress takes time. Look for progress over several weeks or months rather than making decisions about medicine day by day. Stick with my plan to stay with this psychiatrist for at least two years.

Weight gain:

Start a weight control plan now. Start walking in the neighborhood like I used to do. Give up cookies altogether.

Annoyance with doctor:

When I get annoyed, talk to him about it like a grown-up instead of dropping out of treatment. If I have trouble doing it, I can ask my therapist to help.

Too busy:

Make time to help myself. Make myself a higher priority than I have in the past. If I can make time to vacuum, I can make time to work on myself.

No quiet time:

I can find time when I want to. I can go to work a half hour early and sit in the cafeteria where it is quiet, or I can take time on Saturday morning before the kids wake up.

- Ask the doctor to advise you on how to decrease the medications rather than stopping them altogether.
- Decide together how you both will know if symptoms are returning. Perhaps you can keep a Mood Graph (Chapter 4) during the transition.
- Check the Mood Symptoms Worksheet weekly to evaluate your symptoms.
- Promise yourself that you will do what is in your own best interest even if that means admitting that your plan to go off medicines did not work.
- Meet regularly with your doctor or therapist to check your progress.
- If symptoms return, meet with your doctor as soon as possible to decide how to proceed.
- Consider the possibility that even if you can manage without medications at present, it may be necessary to resume them if symptoms return.
- Be certain that going off of medications is worth the risk of relapsing.

What's Next?

One of the most important precautions you can take is to work with your doctor to find a medication regimen that is right for you and stick with it. Most people with bipolar disorder struggle with the idea of taking medication at some point in their lives. So there is a good chance you have already been through it or will find it happening in the future. If you are OK with your medication now, but find yourself having second thoughts about it at a later date, come back and read through this chapter. Perhaps it will help you sort through the issues.

Some clinicians think that when you do not want to take medication you are actually in denial about having bipolar disorder. While this may not always be the reason, it's a possibility. Check out where you are in your adjustment to having bipolar disorder in the next chapter.

chapter seven

Overcoming the Big "D"

In this chapter you will:

✓ Work through your denial about having bipolar disorder.

✓ Learn about the stages of adjusting to a diagnosis of bipolar disorder.

✓ Figure out where you are in the process of adjustment.

✓ Read about how diagnoses of bipolar disorder can be incorrect.

It's very hard to get used to the idea that you have a mental illness that requires treatment, especially when it's first diagnosed. Some people take years to get comfortable enough with the idea even to begin considering treatment. The fact that you're reading this book means you've taken steps toward coping with the idea that you have a mental illness. You have broken through the big "D" of denial.

Denial can take many different forms. It can include disagreeing with or rejecting a diagnosis despite having enough evidence of its existence or refusing to take medications that suggest a specific illness such as refusing lithium because you don't think you have bipolar disorder. Some people with a strong sense of denial would rather tolerate the symptoms and the life disruptions that follow than accept a diagnosis of bipolar disorder and take medication.

Denial can also make you accept the diagnosis, but downplay the seriousness of your illness. It can make you overestimate your ability to cope and underestimate your negative impact on others.

Many people mistakenly assume that if you are no longer in denial about having a mental illness you have achieved acceptance of it and are ready to cooperate with treatment. It's not that simple. Elisabeth Kübler-Ross described the five stages of grief when suffering a loss. These stages include denial, anger, bargaining, depression, and acceptance. When you are diagnosed with bipolar disorder, you may go through similar stages as you grieve the loss of your prior life and accept the challenge of working through your illness and its treatment.

138

Automatic Thoughts and Actions

In Worksheet 7.1 are some examples of the things people say to themselves as they go through each stage of coping with a diagnosis of bipolar disorder. These statements roughly correspond with Kübler-Ross's five stages of adjusting to loss—denial, anger, bargaining, depression, and acceptance. Put a check next to the ones you have experienced in the past and try to identify the stage you may be at right now.

Below each stage is a place for you to write in the thoughts you have had and actions that would have been typical of you as you have gone through each stage of adjustment. Because people can sometimes go backwards in their stage of adjustment, these descriptions may help you recognize when you have lost progress and must work your way toward acceptance again.

Adjustment Is an Ongoing Process

Many people who have bipolar disorder would say they have never fully adjusted to the idea of having a chronic mental illness. They think about it less over time. They resist treatment less. But they never really feel OK about it or reach a point where it doesn't bother them to have to take medications. Acceptance is never complete, but it is possible to get to a point where you can live your life in spite of having bipolar disorder. It may never be exactly the way you had imagined life would be, but that is true for most people. You never know what twists and turns your life will take. It's rare to have all things work out perfectly without hitting bumps along the road. And while it is admittedly much harder for people who must live with a chronic illness, it's possible to adapt, adjust, and come to terms with bipolar disorder and its treatment.

Making peace with yourself for having bipolar disorder **is an ongoing process**. You rarely make your way easily through the stages of grief. There will be gains and setbacks. Anger will reemerge each time the illness interferes with your life, and you will fantasize about the possibility of stopping all your medications and being free of the illness. If you haven't already done so, you will diverge from your path to better mental health, resume bad habits, fall on your face, and then pick yourself up and start over again. Each time you will learn more about how to predict the next fall, what can set you off, and what you need to avoid to stay on a healthy path.

Worksheet 7.2 is a series of questions intended to help you think about your adjustment to having bipolar disorder. Write out your answers in the spaces provided. When you have finished the next section on changing your thinking, come back to what you have written and review your ideas.

worksheet 7.1	**Stages of Adjustment to Bipolar Disorder**

Stage	Automatic thoughts	Actions
Denial	• I don't have it. The doctor made a mistake. • It must be because I've been drinking too much. • The diagnosis is wrong.	• Getting a second opinion. • Looking for other explanations for symptoms. • Ignoring treatment recommendations.
	My thoughts:	*My actions:*
Anger	• It's not fair that I have this illness. • I can't deal with this right now. • Why me? What did I do to deserve this?	• Refusing to listen to advice. • Refusing to discuss the illness. • Losing temper with health care providers, pharmacies, or anyone else associated with treatment.
	My thoughts:	*My actions:*
Bargaining	• I'll clean up my act. • I'll stop drinking, start waking up on time, start exercising, get a better job, and it will be OK. • I'll try natural remedies. I don't really need medicine.	• Adjusting doses on your own. • Changing the timing of doses. • Trading active drugs for "natural remedies." • Staying up late to avoid taking sleeping medications. • Drinking alcohol to reduce anxiety.
	My thoughts:	*My actions:*

worksheet 7.1	**Stages of Adjustment to Bipolar Disorder** (*cont.*)

Depression	• I'll never have a normal life. • No one will want me. • I hate myself.	• Self-destructive behaviors. • Avoidance of doctors, magazine articles, or anything else that reminds you of the illness. • Withdrawal from others.
	My thoughts:	*My actions:*
Acceptance	• I can work my way through this. • It's not the end of the world. • I don't have to give up everything just because I have to take medication.	• Adherence with treatment. • Open discussion of treatment options with clinicians before discontinuing medications.
	My thoughts:	*My actions:*

Couldn't the Diagnosis of Bipolar Disorder Be Wrong?

When people go through denial, one of their biggest questions is about whether they should have received this diagnosis. This concern is a valid one because making a diagnosis of bipolar disorder can be difficult. But even when a diagnosis is correct, acceptance of the diagnosis by patients and their family members is still a challenge.

| **My Thoughts about Having Bipolar Disorder**

Which stage of adjustment are you at right now? How do you know?

What does having bipolar disorder mean to you?

What does it mean about you as a person?

What does it mean about your future?

What effect will it have on the other people in your life?

Are there things you can do to make your future more promising?

Talk these ideas over with your family, friends, doctor, or therapist or with other people who have this illness. As you hear yourself talk about your adjustment to having bipolar, you might work a few things out. After you have read the next chapter on negative thinking, come back to your answers on this worksheet to see if any of the exercises you will learn apply to your thoughts about having the illness.

Diagnostic Challenges

There are two big challenges in making a diagnosis of bipolar disorder, each of which can lead to error and interfere with treatment. The first challenge is timing, the second is accuracy.

Timing

Bipolar disorder looks different depending on when in the course of the illness a diagnosis is made. People with bipolar disorder will be in different states across the course of their lives. There will be periods of depression, periods of mania, and periods of wellness. The periods of illness are called *episodes*. An episode starts with mild symptoms, reaches a peak of severity in the symptoms, and then begins to improve. Therefore, the accuracy of a diagnosis will depend on the clarity and severity of the symptoms. For example, if you were having a major depressive episode, you would look a little tired and a little blue at the beginning of the episode, but eventually reach a low point, called the *nadir*, when the symptoms are at their worst. At the nadir, you might have severe insomnia, be too tired to go to work, feel so hopeless that life does not seem worth living, and find that you no longer care about yourself or others. It would not be unusual at the nadir of an episode to hear voices criticizing you that others cannot hear, to have your eyes play tricks on you to the degree that you see things that other people cannot see, or to become convinced that people are trying to hurt you when there is no real evidence that this is the case. These are called *psychotic symptoms*. They occur when depression is at its worst, but they also occur in psychotic disorders such as schizophrenia or schizoaffective disorder. If a clinician saw you when you were having psychotic symptoms, you might be diagnosed inaccurately as having one of these disorders instead of bipolar disorder.

If you were seen toward the end of an episode of depression, you would look like you did at the beginning of the episode, with milder symptoms, able to function fairly well, but perhaps not yet feeling happy. If you were seen between episodes, when you were no longer having major depression or mania, you would look fine. No one would suspect that you have a mental illness.

The same course applies to mania. At the beginning you would probably look a little hyper, be a little more talkative, and have more self-confidence than usual. It might look like an improvement if you had previously been through an episode of depression. As the symptoms of mania progress and reach their peak you might become agitated, irritable, unable to sit still, and difficult to understand, and you would likely be exercising poor judgment in some way. You might also be grandiose, thinking that you have special powers or that you are more intelligent or gifted than anyone else. At this peak, you might also hear voices telling you to take chances, and you might see visions that you believe are real and have special meaning for you, such as seeing God or angels. These are also called *psychotic symptoms*. If you came into an emergency room talking about your visions and the voices you were hearing and unable to tell about your history of depression and mania, you would very likely be mistaken as having a psychotic disorder like schizophrenia or schizoaffective disorder. If you had also been using street drugs or drinking alcohol, someone might think your symptoms were just a sign of a severe substance abuse problem.

Some people come down from the high of mania and plunge into an episode of depression rather than returning to their normal self. An episode of mania can leave you feeling exhausted, out of sorts, disoriented, and unable to function well on your own. If you were seen at this point and your history was not apparent, it might be hard to know if you were ending a mania or in the middle of a depression.

Another complexity related to timing is the age at which the symptoms began. In adults, mania and depression are fairly easy to distinguish from normal states. Manias are often euphoric, and the person feels better than good. Depressions make people feel sad or tearful. When bipolar disorder begins in childhood or during adolescence, the picture is not as clear. Kids are more likely to feel irritable and angry than sad or euphoric. Also, kids are not as able as adults to verbalize feeling states. They know that they feel bad, but they may not be able to be more specific. Children do not have the coping abilities of adults, so when they feel bad they may act up in ways that looks like misbehavior. They may be argumentative, defiant, uncompromising, rascally, and impulsive in much the same way that kids do who have conduct disorder problems, hyperactivity, or attention deficit disorder. If you were diagnosed early in life, it is likely that you would be given one of these more common childhood diagnoses and treated accordingly.

Another timing concern is in the progression of the illness. Suppose that in the early phases of your illness you had two episodes of major depression before you ever had your first manic episode. Let's say the first episode occurred at age 16 years, when your parents divorced. You may have gotten some therapy, or it may have passed on its own, but it would not have been accurate to diagnose you with bipolar disorder after just one episode of depression. Depending on the length and severity of the depression, it would have been called either *bereavement* or *major depression*.

If you had another episode of depression when you finished high school and were heading to college or your first job, most people would have said that it was just stress because you were not sure where you were going in life or were afraid to be on your own. You probably would have not sought treatment unless the symptoms caused you to drop out of school or get fired from your job. At that point, the correct diagnosis for you would have been *recurrent major depression*. However, if you had been like many people who had figured out that alcohol or street drugs made them feel better temporarily when depressed, the diagnostic picture would have been even more confusing. When depression and alcohol or substance abuse occur at the same time, it is very difficult to tell which caused which. When you had your first manic episode, however, your diagnosis would have been changed from recurrent major depression to *bipolar disorder.*

In this example, the correct diagnosis changed as the illness progressed. The initial diagnosis of major depression would have been correct because mania had not yet occurred and no one could have known that mania was coming. The fact that the diagnosis was changed to bipolar disorder after mania happened for the first time does not mean that the first diagnosis of major depression was wrong. It had been correct at the time it was given. After a diagnosis of bipolar disorder is given, the old diagnosis of recurrent major depression no longer applies. If asked, you would not tell someone that you used to have recurrent depression and now you have bipolar disorder, nor would you say that you have both. Instead, the diagnosis of bipolar disorder becomes your primary diagnosis. Doctors understand that when you have bipolar disorder you will have periods of depression as well as periods of mania, hypomania, and mixed states.

The point of explaining how these complications can interfere with a correct diagnosis is to help you understand how the diagnostic process can be challenging. If you think that the timing of your symptoms might have led clinicians to draw the wrong conclusion about you, ask your doctor to explain why he or she thinks you have bipolar disorder or get another clinical opinion on your diagnosis. Rather than reject a diagnosis, get more information about it.

Accuracy

Research studies on the accuracy of diagnoses made by clinicians consistently show that errors can be made. Despite advances in other areas of medicine, psychiatry, which deals with the most complex organ, the brain, does not yet have the technology to accurately detect physical indicators of specific illnesses such as bipolar disorder. Because there are no current laboratory tests that can confirm the existence of mental illnesses in individuals, all diagnoses are made by reviewing the person's symptoms and determining whether the pattern meets the DSM-IV-TR criteria discussed in Chapter 2. Making a correct judgment depends on the amount of information available to the clinician as well as the thoroughness of the clinician and his or her level of training and skill. With so many variables at work, there is a lot of room for error.

Mistakes in diagnoses are made most often for two reasons: (1) the patient is not able to provide enough information on his or her history and progression of symptoms to aid diagnosis, and (2) several different psychological or medical problems can occur simultaneously, such as depression and alcohol use or mania and cocaine use or mood symptoms and psychotic symptoms. Adding to the complexity of the picture are cultural, language, and geographic differences in the way symptoms appear. For example, what looks like hypomania in west Texas may look normal in southern California. In some cultures, psychological distress is more likely to be experienced as physical symptoms, while in others it is expressed as emotion. Patients with limited English-speaking skills may have trouble communicating with clinicians who do not understand their native language. Or the culture of the clinician may cause him or her to misinterpret signs and symptoms in someone from a different culture.

Research studies show that the most accurate psychiatric diagnoses are those made using structured diagnostic interviews. Unfortunately, those methods are usually available only in research clinics or clinics affiliated with medical schools and rarely in general psychiatric practices.

Accuracy can be a very real problem in diagnosing bipolar disorder. However, if you've been diagnosed by several different clinicians as having bipolar disorder and you have experienced the symptoms described in Chapters 1 through 4, there is a good chance that your diagnosis is accurate. If, despite a lot of evidence, you are still fighting the diagnosis, maybe it's time to reexamine the facts and take charge of your mood swings.

Acceptance

Inability to accept a diagnosis usually means unwillingness to participate fully in the assessment process and in treatment. It is one thing to understand what a doctor means when he or she says that you have bipolar disorder. It's another to find it acceptable and believable. Agreeing with a diagnosis of bipolar disorder means accepting not only that you have a mental illness, but also that you have one that will require lifelong treatment. This is a lot to swallow at one time. It is natural to resist the idea, say that the doctor is wrong, explain away the symptoms as due to stress or too much partying, or believe that you're just going through a phase. If you do not want to be given a diagnosis of bipolar disorder, you might not be completely honest with the doctor about your symptoms. You might downplay mood swings and changes in your behavior that occurred when manic or depressed. In this case, your lack of acceptance can interfere with the diagnostic process. And if you know that you have been less than completely forthright in the information you have given and the diagnosis still comes out to be bipolar disorder, you will question the accuracy of the diagnosis.

Doesn't Everyone Have Mood Swings?

Mood swings vary greatly in severity, as the figure at the bottom of the page shows. On the low end of severity is the normal range of human experience, where people feel down when bad things happen and feel elated when good things happen. These states are usually temporary and relate specifically to an event. When the event is over, the mood returns to normal or neutral. There are also some people who are moody by nature. They do not have the physical symptoms of depression or mania; they are just cranky or temperamental. They do not have a mental illness, but they are different from the happy-go-lucky type. Then there are those who are perky, optimistic, and hopeful, even in the face of adversity. They are not manic, just good-natured.

Moving up the scale in severity are people whose mood is worsened by physical problems or stress. The best example is premenstrual syndrome, or PMS. Women who have PMS have a definite drop in their mood that can last a week or so prior to starting their periods and can linger for a few days afterward. It is caused by changes in hormone levels, bloating, pain, and other physical discomforts, but it goes away as predictably as it arrives. Low blood sugar can also cause moodiness for anyone but is more severe in those who have diabetes. Seasonal allergy attacks can cause irritability until symptoms subside, as can other physical discomforts such as rashes or pain. Stress alters mood, causing irritability, anxiety, sadness, and frustration. If the stressful problem persists, the negative mood state persists. Stress can cause some of the symptoms of bipolar disorder, such as irritability and insomnia, in people who do not have the illness.

More severe are the diagnosable mood disorders. *Diagnosable* means that they meet criteria set out in the DSM-IV-TR. Dysthymia or dysthymic disorder is a chronic but usually mild depression that can be lifelong. It is more than being moody, but not as severe as major depression. In dysthymia, people have a low mood at least half the time and a few of the physical features of major depression or low self-esteem. People who have dysthymia can also have periods of major depres-

None/Low		Moderate		Severe	
Normal	Moody Perky	PMS Allergies Stressed Low blood sugar	Cyclothymia Dysthymia Minor depression	Bipolar II Major depression	Bipolar I

Range of severity of mood swings.

sion during the course of their life. When their major depression is over, they usually go back to being dysthymic.

Cyclothymia is a mild form of bipolar disorder and is also lifelong. There are ups that look like hypomania and downs that are fairly mild that alternate throughout a person's life. What looks like cyclothymia could also be the beginnings of the development of bipolar disorder.

Minor depression is also called *depression NOS* (not otherwise specified) and is diagnosed when a person has a sad mood and a few of the physical symptoms listed under major depression, but falls short of the five symptoms needed to diagnose major depression. Minor depression is often triggered by a stressful event, lasts for a short while until the person gets over the event, and usually remits without treatment.

Bipolar II and major depression vary greatly in severity, and although they are listed on the continuum as less severe than bipolar I disorder, they can be just as chronic and cause just as much misery. Major depression has already been described. Once it occurs, it tends to recur, sometimes related to distressing events and sometimes for no reason at all. It can also be chronic, lasting years at a time with no relief.

Bipolar II disorder is defined as having periods of major depression and periods of hypomania. Hypomania, as mentioned earlier, is different from mania only by degree. It includes the changes in mood, thought, and physical symptoms of mania but does not impair judgment so much that a person gets into trouble.

Moving higher on the continuum past bipolar I disorder are schizoaffective disorder, bipolar type, and schizophrenia with bipolar NOS. With both of these illnesses there is usually no time of wellness. When the manias or depressions subside, psychotic symptoms such as hallucinations and delusions usually continue to persist. The difference between these two disorders is that in schizoaffective disorder, bipolar type, the person has episodes of depression and mania as often as someone who has bipolar I disorder. In schizophrenia, the episodes of mania and depression occur much less frequently and do not last as long as they would in the bipolar I or schizoaffective disorders.

Now that you have read about the many different types of mood swings, you may be able to better understand why your doctor and therapists think you have bipolar disorder instead of just run-of-the-mill mood changes. If you think your symptoms would be better explained as a different disorder, talk it over with your doctor or therapist.

▶ What's Next?

You have now completed the chapters in this workbook on taking precautions to prevent future episodes of mania and depression. In the next set of chapters you will advance to Step 3 in the CBT approach to bipolar disorder and learn methods to reduce your symptoms when they are present.

If you go back to Chapter 1 and review the CBT model of bipolar disorder, you will find changes in cognition and emotion near the top of the cycle where depression and mania begin. Cognitions or thoughts have a strong influence on your emotions and your behavioral reactions. Therefore, methods for catching, controlling, and correcting distorted or overly emotional thoughts will be covered in Chapters 8 and 9. You can learn to recognize when your mood is being colored by your thinking and sort out your emotional and logical thoughts before you overreact to them.

Step 3

Reduce Your Symptoms

chapter eight

Recognizing and Catching Your Thinking Errors

In this chapter you will:

✓ Figure out how your mood can affect your thoughts and reactions to events.

✓ Review the ways in which your thoughts can become distorted or inaccurate.

✓ Learn the *catch it, control it, correct it* method for straightening out distorted thinking.

Bipolar disorder produces strong emotions such as sadness, irritability, excitement, anxiety, and anger during episodes of depression and mania and sometimes between episodes as well. These emotions or moods can make you more prone to overreact to upsetting situations.

For example, when Amanda is depressed, she is more easily overwhelmed when there is too much to do. Last week Amanda's son told her on Sunday afternoon that he had a project due at school the next morning and he needed some supplies from the store. Amanda already had plenty of chores to do that day and resented this last-minute announcement. When she found out that the assignment had been given 2 weeks before, she could feel her blood boil. Even though her son was just a middle schooler, she got angry and complained that he was irresponsible, inconsiderate, and unappreciative of how hard she works. He apologized and went to his room. After she calmed down, she felt bad about yelling at him, so she put aside her chores, took him to the store, and helped him with his project. When Amanda is not depressed, she still doesn't like things to upset her schedule, but she doesn't usually overreact and yell at her kids over small things.

Have you ever found yourself in a similar situation? Take a moment and write down on Worksheet 8.1 a recent event that upset you, the thoughts that went through your head when it first occurred, and how you reacted to the situation.

worksheet 8.1	**Events, Thoughts, and Actions—Pressured Situation**

The event	Your thoughts	How you handled it
Amanda's example: My son told me at the last minute that he had a project to do.	*He's irresponsible. He is inconsiderate. He does not appreciate how hard I work and how much I have to do.*	*Yelled at my son and made him feel bad. Later felt bad. Took him to the store and helped him with his project.*
Your example:		

From *The Bipolar Workbook* by Monica Ramirez Basco. Copyright 2006 by The Guilford Press. Permission to photocopy this form is granted to purchasers of this book for personal use only (see copyright page for details).

Your mood sets you up to overreact, but what determines your emotional response to events is what you think about the situation. Amanda was in a bad mood to start with, but the reason she reacted so strongly to her son was that she thought his request meant that he did not value her time and how hard she worked, because if he did value her time he would not drop things on her at the last minute. In this situation Amanda thought the issue was about her when it was actually about a kid who forgot to do his homework project.

It's easy to see how external events can trigger an emotional reaction like the one Amanda had toward her son. But as described in the first chapter, the emotional changes that occur during periods of depression and mania can stir up emotional thoughts even when nothing in particular is happening. Here is another example from Amanda.

Amanda's depression makes her feel down and doubt that things will ever get better. The more she thinks about her problems, the more hopeless she feels. She says things to herself like "I can't believe my life is such a mess. I'm never going to get out of debt. I can't keep up with this house and the kids and my job. I may as well just give up." If she starts thinking this way when she wakes up in the morning, she feels no motivation to get out of bed, to interact with the family, or to pay her bills, even though she knows they are overdue. Amanda's depression affects her thoughts, making them negative and hopeless. Both her bad mood and her dark thoughts take away her motivation to get up and take on another day. She stays in bed, lets her husband tend to the kids, and leaves the bills on her desk for another day.

If you've been in a similar situation, describe it in the boxes on Worksheet 8.2.

Amanda's examples have shown how your mood can affect your thoughts and your choice of actions during periods of depression, but the same thing can happen during periods of mania. During his last two manic episodes, Tommy felt euphoric for a while, but later became irritable and angry. Here is an example of the type of thing that would occur.

| worksheet 8.2 | **Events, Thoughts, and Actions—Worry** |

The event	Your thoughts	How you handled it
Amanda's example: Woke up and started thinking about my problems.	I can't believe my life is such a mess. I'm never going to get out of debt. I can't keep up with this house and the kids and my job. I may as well just give up.	Stayed in bed. Let my husband tend to the kids. Left the bills on my desk for another day.
Your example:		

Tommy was feeling edgy when he walked into his parents' house to have dinner with them. His mother noticed that Tommy was pacing around a lot more than usual and asked him if he had taken his medication. Tommy blew up at her. "Get off my case about the medicine. I hate taking that stuff. You're always badgering me about it. Why do you have to make me angry? Can't we get through one evening without you bringing that up again? I'm leaving." Tommy went out the door and slammed it behind him, got in his car, and sped away. He went to a friend's house and drank a few beers until he calmed down enough to go back to his apartment.

Tommy's irritability set him up to overreact to his mother's question, but what led to his outburst was that he thought his mother was trying to badger him and make him angry. He did not think that she was showing concern. He thought she was getting on his case about taking medicines. Tommy was too angry to talk it over with her, so he left. This is another good example of how your thoughts about a situation can determine your reaction to it. If you have ever been in a situation like Tommy's when your irritability made you overreact, jot it down on Worksheet 8.3.

| worksheet 8.3 | **Events, Thoughts, and Actions—Medication Issue** |

The event	Your thoughts	How you handled it
Tommy's example: My mom asked me if I'd taken my medication.	She's on my case. She is badgering me. She knows I hate taking medications and she still brings it up.	Yelled at my mom. Left without eating dinner. Sped off in my car. Drank beer until I calmed down.
Your example:		

As with depression, mania can produce spontaneous thoughts that arouse emotions, like having a great idea all of a sudden and feeling good about it. There may have been triggers in your environment that inspired you, but you may not have been aware of them. Spontaneous creative thoughts or ideas can be very exciting and make you want to pursue them even if it isn't practical at the time.

Paul is a creative person. When he's becoming manic, however, he tends to have a lot more ideas and inspirations. As he was watching television one evening just before bedtime, he saw a commercial about a new reading program for kids who had difficulty in school. He remembered how much trouble he had had reading as a kid and had a wonderful idea for a program that would be so much better than the one in the commercial. Paul got out of bed and went to his computer to write down his ideas. At 3:00 A.M. Paul noticed that he was getting tired and remembered that he had to be at work by 8:00 a.m. He knew himself fairly well and recognized what he had been doing for the last three hours as a manic burst of energy. He knew that if he stayed up all night and worked on his project he would get more manic. He looked at the pillbox sitting on his nightstand and realized that he had not taken his medication earlier. Taking it now would make him sleep through the alarm, so he turned off the computer and tried to sleep without it. After tossing and turning for some time he was able to fall asleep for a few hours before the alarm went off.

Paul's new idea may have been an excellent one and worthy of his time. The problem was not the project. The problem was the timing. Going with his spontaneous idea made him forget his evening medication and kept him up much later than he could afford. The end result was that the next day Paul was exhausted at work, but his mind was beginning to race, a symptom that mania was coming.

Think of a time when you might have had an experience like Paul's and write about it on Worksheet 8.4. Try to remember how you felt compelled to take action right away rather than wait for a time that was more convenient. Mania can make you think that things are more urgent than they really are and that if you don't take action right away you will lose your wonderful idea altogether. The actions taken can create new problems if they disrupt your sleep and make you forget to take your medication.

Each of the examples provided shows how emotions can set you up to overreact to internal or external events. Your reactions are based on your evaluation of the situation—that is, what you think about it. As illustrated, the thoughts fueled by depression or mania can be distorted by emotions. They can be overly negative or overly positive, depending on your mood. The bigger problem is that your emotional reactions and what you think about a situation will dictate how well you handle it. If you're not seeing things accurately, you're not always going to handle the situation well.

worksheet 8.4	**Events, Thoughts and Actions—Creative Ideas**

The event	Your thoughts	How you handled it
Paul's example: Saw a TV commercial that stimulated a creative idea about a reading program.	I have a great idea. It's so much better than the one on TV. I better work on it right now, before I lose the idea. This is going to make me a lot of money.	Got out of bed. Didn't take evening medications. Worked at the computer until 3:00 A.M. Slept for only a few hours before having to go to work.
Your example:		

From *The Bipolar Workbook* by Monica Ramirez Basco. Copyright 2006 by The Guilford Press. Permission to photocopy this form is granted to purchasers of this book for personal use only (see copyright page for details).

The Triple-C Method for Controlling Your Thoughts

The exercises in this chapter and the next are aimed at helping you recognize when your mood or emotions are distorting your perceptions. If you can catch overly emotional thinking when it occurs, you can take control of it rather than letting it control your reactions. One way to do this is to become aware of when you are thinking in an overly emotional way. If you can catch it happening, you have a chance to control it. One way of controlling your reactions is to choose a course of action that would be better for you, and another is to correct your emotional thinking so that it does not lead you in the wrong direction.

Catch   the distortions in thinking when they occur.

Control   them by keeping them from influencing your behavior.

Correct   any errors in your logic.

To catch distorted thinking you have to know what to look for. There are some common patterns in the ways depression and mania can color your thinking. They are called *thinking errors*. The following pages describe some of the more common thinking errors people make when depressed and when manic. If you can catch yourself making any of these thinking errors, you will have an opportunity to correct the distortions before they lead you in the wrong direction. The most common thinking errors in depression and mania fall into four categories:

1. **Misperceptions,** which include magnification and minimization.
2. **Jumping to conclusions,** which includes mind reading, fortune telling, catastrophizing, and personalization.
3. **Tunnel vision,** sometimes called selective perception or mental filtering.
4. **Absolutes,** which include black-and-white thinking, labeling, and shoulds.

In the rest of this chapter you'll read descriptions of each of the four thinking error categories, with examples of the forms they might take during periods of depression and during periods of mania. As you read, try to recall times when you might have made each thinking error in response to a stressful situation. Worksheets in which you can record your personal examples will be provided throughout. Also in this chapter are methods for controlling these thinking errors. In the next chapter, you'll find exercises aimed at the third C—correcting distortions in thinking whenever they occur. Practice these methods for controlling and correcting thinking errors and you'll find over time that they will be less likely to occur and, when they do occur, you'll be able to correct or dismiss them quickly.

CATCH IT!

Misperceptions

Misperceptions occur when existing information is distorted, making it GREATER or SMALLER than it really is. Worksheets 8.5 and 8.6 provide examples of misperceptions in depression and mania, respectively. Think of times when you misperceived a situation by either magnifying or minimizing the facts and enter your examples in the spaces provided in the worksheets.

| worksheet 8.5 | **Misperceptions in Depression** |

Misperception	Amanda's examples	My examples
Magnification of the seriousness of problems	*This is so horrible. I'll never forgive myself for forgetting my mom's birthday.*	
Minimization of positive events or accomplishments OR Dismissing compliments	*It doesn't matter that I finally got the kitchen clean. I should never have let it get this bad.* Amanda's boss: *You did a good job!* Amanda minimizes: *It's no big deal.* Amanda: *Your report card looks pretty good!* Her daughter minimizes: *Yeah, whatever.*	

CONTROL IT!

Magnification

In depression and mania, magnification is fueled by the emotion of the moment. When the intensity of the emotion decreases, magnification tends to diminish. For example, if you're angry, an upsetting situation may seem intolerable; once you've calmed down, however, the situation may seem bothersome but manageable. If you're feeling sad and are left out by a group of friends, you might feel devastated at first, but after you are able to calm down you might feel hurt yet able to deal with it. Emotions that fuel magnification can be lessened by gaining emotional distance from an event or idea, allowing you time to think before you react.

Some common ways of gaining emotional distance are:

- Walk away from the situation.
- Take time to evaluate it.
- Ask others for their opinion of the event.
- Sleep on it.
- Compare the event that is magnified to other experiences you have had.
- Ask yourself how others might view what happened.
- Hold your breath and count to ten before you react.

| worksheet 8.6 | **Misperceptions in Mania** |

Misperception	Paul's examples	My examples
Magnification in self-esteem or in the value of ideas	*This plan can't possibly fail. This is the best idea anyone has had in a long time. This is pure genius.*	
Minimization of the seriousness of problems or risks	Paul's girlfriend: *Slow down!!* Paul minimizes: *It's OK. I've never gotten a speeding ticket on <u>this</u> highway.*	

- Watch television for a while.
- Change the subject.
- Meditate.
- Take a nap.
- Refuse to talk about it until you've calmed down.

When you are upset, how do you gain emotional distance? Write down your ideas and experiences on Worksheet 8.7.

Paul gains emotional distance from his manic ideas by talking them over with his friends. For example, Paul talked to his friends at work about his reading program idea. After hearing their input he was not as convinced that it was the most wonderful idea he had ever had and that it was guaranteed to succeed. In fact, the more he talked to them about it, the less enthusiastic Paul felt about working on the idea. Knowing himself and his tendency to get caught up in his own fantasies, he dismissed the idea as a manic thought and focused on his current work and school responsibilities.

CONTROL IT!

Minimization

Minimization occurs during both episodes of depression and episodes of mania. When depressed, you might use minimization to push away information that is inconsistent with your negative mood, for example, pushing away compliments or

worksheet 8.7	**Gaining Emotional Distance**

I gain emotional distance by:

praise. When in a manic state, you might use minimization to push away anything that is contrary to your positive mood or great ideas. This can take the form of ignoring possible risks, like spending more money than you can afford, driving too fast, or being more sexually active than usual. When you minimize positives or negatives, you distort available information to make it fit your state of mind and mood. When you distort information and can't see things clearly, you can easily make mistakes.

Minimizing Negatives

When entering a manic phase, you're susceptible to minimizing negatives. For example, you might overlook important details such as risks or disadvantages of situations. When you minimize negatives, the positive aspects of any idea can seem even more outstanding. You can convince yourself that there is no down side or that the risks are small and the benefits great even if this is not true.

To avoid minimizing, ask yourself and others the following questions:

- **What is the down side to my idea or plan?**
- **Are any risks involved?**
- **Could I be overlooking something important?**
- **Am I disregarding or ignoring important facts?**

Make yourself look at all the angles before drawing your conclusions and taking action.

If Paul were going to use this strategy to sort out his thoughts about the new reading program he was inventing, he would answer these questions as follows:

- **What is the down side to my idea or plan?** *It will take a lot of time to work out the details of the program, and it may interfere with my other goals or with my sleep.*

- **Are any risks involved?** *If I put money into this plan, I could lose it if the idea is a flop. If I keep staying up late at night to work on it, I will probably get manic. I don't want to get manic again.*

- **Could I be overlooking something important?** *This could be just another of my manic fantasies that turns out to be a bad idea. I've been through times like this before.*

- **Am I disregarding or ignoring important facts?** *I don't know much about helping kids to read other than my own personal experience. I'm not sure what facts I'm overlooking.*

Minimizing Positives

When you're not depressed, you might minimize positives or dismiss compliments as an act of humility or modesty. In those situations, pushing away praise is a social behavior, but in your heart you still feel good about the compliment. For example, if someone pays you a compliment on your cooking by saying, "That is the best pie I've ever had," you might minimize it by saying, "Oh, it's not that great. The crust should have been a little lighter." When in a depressed or irritable state, you minimize positives because you don't think they count. You might think you're not worthy of praise or your actions are too inadequate to matter. Some common ways in which people minimize positives are:

- Discounting successes because they are not good enough
- Disqualifying a positive thought with a negative thought
- Dismissing compliments

Minimizing positives is particularly a problem for people who have extremely high expectations or who are perfectionists. Nothing is good enough unless it is perfect. With this train of thought you are not able to enjoy the small accomplishments that build up to become bigger accomplishments. For example, you may have finished writing a term paper but don't feel good about it because you had to stay up all night to do it. You tell yourself it should have been done sooner. Instead of feeling joy and relief, you feel guilt and disappointment. Negative emotions like these feed depression.

When you're in a bad mood and think that nothing is going your way, you might minimize or completely ignore evidence to the contrary. For example, if you were in a bad mood and you were lucky enough to get a good parking space, you might minimize the positive by thinking, "So what? My car is old, falling apart, and I can't afford a new one." If you are a student and do well on a test, you might push away the accomplishment by thinking, "I still have a lot of work to do, and there's no guarantee I'll do well on the next test." If you are shopping and find a bargain, you might minimize it by thinking, "I have to buy things on sale. I don't have a lot of money like other people who are paying full price."

Some people minimize positives even when they are not depressed. They can always think of the down side, why things won't work, or what could spoil a positive event. We call them pessimists. Their glass is always half empty. If you are a pessimist by nature and you have bipolar disorder, you're likely to bring yourself down during depressed phases by minimizing positives and not allowing yourself the small joys of accomplishment that could lift your spirits.

To control minimizing, you can use a method called **thought stopping**. This is a strategy that was developed for the treatment of rumination or obsessive thoughts. Its goal is to stop minimization and replace it with something more accurate. **Thought stopping to control minimization involves three steps:**

The first step is to catch yourself doing it. That's the hardest part. It can help to enlist the assistance of someone in your family or a friend to alert you when he or she hears you minimize. Try to pay attention to situations where you become aware of a positive and then push it away. There are probably patterns that you can come to recognize. Maybe your minimization takes the form of dismissing praise, for example. If so, you can watch for it when receiving positive feedback from others. If your pattern is to disqualify things you've accomplished, you probably minimize on a regular basis. As you get things done, listen to that voice in your head that tells you it doesn't count, doesn't matter, or isn't worth mentioning. It can help to keep a log of the types of things you minimize so you can learn to catch yourself in the act of minimizing.

The second step, once you have caught yourself minimizing, is to control the thought by telling yourself in a commanding voice to "STOP!" Practice telling yourself to stop out loud or in your head. Find a tone of voice that sounds like an authority, like a parent. "Stop that!" "Stop that right now!" "Cut that out!" "That's enough!" "Quit it!" Think about how you would tell someone else in a strong voice to stop what they were doing. Use that tone on yourself when you catch yourself minimizing your positives.

The third step in thought stopping is to switch the thought to something more positive. If you catch yourself about to dismiss a compliment from someone, tell yourself to "STOP!" and say "Thank you" instead. If you catch yourself minimizing your accomplishments, like getting some work done that might have been hard for you, tell yourself that it's OK to feel good about it. Try statements like "At least I got something done" or "It may be a small accomplishment, but it's still positive" or "When I'm feeling this bad, anything I can do is a good thing." You will have to find a thought to replace your minimization. The most helpful ones are those that allow you to see your positives for what they are.

Raquel had a bad habit of pushing away praise and telling herself that even when she did do something right, it was never good enough. She learned to use thought stopping to control her minimization. The most common example for Raquel is that when someone thanks her or praises her she follows their compliment with a self-criticism. For example, an interaction with her husband early in their marriage might have sounded like this:

HUSBAND: *Thanks for dinner. It was really good.* [praise]

RAQUEL: *It was a little underdone.* [self-criticism]

HUSBAND: *I still like it.* [praise]

RAQUEL: *You're easy to please.* [discounted his praise]

The end result of many conversations like this was that compliments were delivered, but never received by Raquel. Therefore, they had no positive impact on her. Rejection of his praises, however, frustrated Raquel's husband, so after a while he learned not to offer them anymore. Raquel noticed at some point that her husband had stopped praising her. Her interpretation was that her cooking really wasn't good enough and her husband had stopped pretending that it was. One Thanksgiving she worked particularly hard to provide a memorable meal. Raquel received praise from everyone except her husband. She took offense and acted cold toward him until he implored her to tell him what he had done wrong. When she told him what had upset her, he explained that he loved her cooking but had given up praising her for it because she always disagreed with him and pushed away the compliment. He found it hurtful, so he stopped doing it. Raquel knew that she tended to minimize positives and vowed to learn to accept praise. Now when she hears her husband say that he has enjoyed dinner she tells herself to "STOP!" before the negative remark leaves her lips and just say "Thank you. I'm glad you enjoyed it."

CATCH IT!

Jumping to Conclusions

Jumping to conclusions is a thinking error that occurs when people make guesses or assumptions before knowing all the facts. You can jump to conclusions by making guesses or assumptions about people or about events. In general, if you're feeling depressed, the guesses are usually negative or upsetting. If you're manic and feeling euphoric, your guesses are likely to be overly positive. If you're irritable, your guesses will stir up your anger. The conclusions you jump to usually match your mood. If you're anxious, you'll predict scary things. If you're jealous, you'll see betrayal even when it's not there. If you're angry, you'll assume that others have negative intentions. The problem with jumping to conclusions is that they are often incorrect. When you act on them, you make mistakes. There are many different ways in which we jump to conclusions. As each is described, think of times when you may have thought the same way and later found out you were wrong. Jot down some of your own examples in the worksheets.

> **Mind reading: Guessing what others are thinking or how they are feeling** *(Worksheet 8.8).*

Manic Mike: *I know she's interested in me. She probably wore that dress just to get my attention.*

Nervous Nellie: *I can tell he's mad at me.*

Depressed Doris: *They probably think it's my fault that it didn't work out.*

Hypomanic Hillary: *They are just jealous because the teacher likes me best.*

Worried Wanda: *He's acting funny today. I don't think he likes me anymore.*

---

worksheet 8.8 | **Mind Reading**

My own examples of mind reading:

> **Fortune telling: Making predictions about future events** *(Worksheet 8.9).*

Down-Hearted Donald: *It's not going to work out. Nothing works out for me.*

Hypomanic Harriett: *Once she hears this idea for making the office more efficient, I know she'll give me a raise, maybe even a promotion. I should be in charge. So what if I'm new on the job?*

Anxious Annie: *I'm going to make a fool of myself. I'll probably forget what I'm supposed to say and stand there staring at them like an idiot.*

Overconfident Oscar: *I just know I can ace that test without even having to open a book.*

worksheet 8.9	**Fortune Telling**

My own examples of fortune telling:

***Catastrophizing: Assuming the worst-case scenario is likely to happen** (Worksheet 8.10).*

Stressed-Out Sally: *If my car repairs are too expensive, I'm not going to have enough money to pay my rent this month. I'm going to get evicted. I'll have to live in the streets.*

Down-in-the-Dumps Darla: *I'm never going to get this paper finished in time. I'm going to end up failing the class and not graduating.*

Irritable Irene: *This is going to take all day. I don't have time for this. We picked the wrong line to stand in. I'm going to miss my flight.*

***Personalization: Assuming that events are all about you without knowing all the facts; taking things personally** (Worksheet 8.11).*

Discouraged Denise: *It's my fault my son is in so much trouble at school. If only I had been a better mother.*

Hyper Harvey: *Did you see how they looked at me when we walked in? They stopped talking for a second just to see what I would do next.*

| worksheet 8.10 | **Catastrophizing** |

My own examples of catastrophizing:

| worksheet 8.11 | **Personalization** |

My own examples of personalization:

CONTROL IT!

How *Not* to Jump to Conclusions

When you jump to conclusions, you're making guesses or assumptions about a situation, a problem, or a person. You might be convinced that your assumption is correct, but if emotion is influencing your thinking, there's a good chance that you could be wrong. To avoid making mistakes, you have to consider other likely explanations for what is happening to you or around you and choose the option that makes the most sense. If you're not sure how to interpret the words or actions of others, ask for additional information or check out your assumptions before you draw your conclusion. When you're not upset, you probably do this automatically. When you're filled with strong emotions or when situations stimulate strong reactions in you, you may need to pause long enough to think things through more logically before you draw an accurate conclusion. Some guidelines will be provided in the following sections for how to control the more common forms of jumping to conclusions.

Mind Reading

When you're depressed, anxious, or irritable, your mood will make you jump to negative conclusions about what people are thinking or feeling. You can easily convince yourself that you're right by thinking of evidence that supports your conclusion and ignoring all other opposing evidence. Mind reading is based on the assumption that if you know someone well enough, you know how he or she feels or what he or she thinks about most situations. What gives you confidence to mind read is that occasionally you are right. Mind reading is a problem when the conclusions you jump to are incorrect but you act as if they are true. When your instincts are wrong, the actions that follow can cause you more distress and create problems with other people.

Mind reading is a common cause of arguments among people. If you're feeling irritable, it's easy to find yourself making negative assumptions about people rather than asking questions. Some common mind-reading statements that are prone to fuel an argument are as follows:

- *I know what you're thinking.*
- *You know I'm right.*
- *I know you better than you know yourself.*
- *I can tell you're mad.*
- *You think you're smarter than everyone else.*
- *You think you're perfect.*

No matter who you're talking to, these are the kinds of words that can start a fight. **The way to avoid mind reading and the conflict it can cause is to ask questions instead of making mind-reading statements.** Here are some alternatives to consider:

- *What are you thinking?*
- *Do you agree with me?*
- *Because I know you pretty well, I would bet that you are feeling. . . . Am I right?*
- *Are you mad?*
- *I sometimes get the impression that you think you're smarter than me, and that really bothers me.*
- *You may not realize this, but when you criticize me it's as if you're saying that you're perfect and I'm messed up. Is that what you think?*

Fortune Telling

To avoid fortune-telling errors, it's helpful to remember that just because your guess about what will happen next stirs up a lot of emotion does not mean that it's correct. A lot of people think their first thoughts reflect their instincts about a situation. If you think your instincts can be trusted when you're upset, you will latch on to the first ideas that come to mind. However, just because it was the first thing you thought of does not mean that it's right. In fact, your first thoughts in reaction to a stressful event are usually full of emotion, and emotions can distort your thinking. If you jump to the conclusion that something bad is going to happen and act on this first impression, you could easily be going down the wrong path.

The solution to fortune telling is to consider other possible outcomes rather than stop at your first guess.

Raquel and her boss have had a rocky relationship for many years. She admits to being overly sensitive when it comes to dealing with him. But there have been times in the past when he has taken advantage of her willingness to work hard or tried to cheat her on her salary or vacation pay. When she has to interact with him, she can't help feeling a little defensive. Feeling defensive can sometimes make her jump to conclusions about what he tells her. For example, he called her into his office to tell her that sales have been down this month and some changes would have to be made. She immediately thought, "We're not going to get the raises we were promised or the overtime pay. This company does not care about its employees. It only cares about the bottom line. I should just quit." Before she said anything, her boss went on to explain that they were going to change their product line and make less of the low-profit items and more of the higher-profit items. That would mean that Raquel needed to make some changes to the orders she had placed earlier that week.

Even though Raquel heard the instructions, she kept waiting for the other shoe to drop. She had not yet considered the possibility that she had jumped to conclusions. She was sure that bad news was coming. She left her boss's office but did not lower her guard. She stayed tense for weeks as they worked through the production changes, waiting for her boss to deliver the bad news. As it turned out, Raquel was wrong, and she had spent several stressful weeks waiting for her initial incorrect predictions to come to pass.

When you can catch yourself jumping to conclusions in response to a stressful situation, consider the other possible outcomes that could occur rather than stopping at the first one that comes to mind. Raquel, for example, could have also considered the possibility that her boss was telling the truth or that she was only partially right about the consequences. **When you are uncertain about what will happen next in a stressful situation, try to get more information.** Raquel could have saved herself a lot of worry if she had asked the boss directly about the raises and overtime pay. If he had bad news, as Raquel imagined, instead of spending several weeks worrying she could have used the time to find a better solution or a way to cope with her circumstances.

Catastrophizing

Catastrophizing is an extreme version of fortune telling where you jump to the conclusion that is the worst possible outcome. Catastrophizing is fueled by anxiety and worry. Allowing yourself to believe that a catastrophe will occur usually makes your anxiety worse. When you're in this state, you panic and feel helpless to change the course of events. Not everyone catastrophizes when worried, but those who do tend to find that it's a common occurrence for them. If this sounds like you, there are some things you can do to stop the panic and take control over the situation.

Raquel has a tendency to catastrophize when stressed out. This year it was her turn to have her husband's family at the house for Christmas. She and her husband had managed to avoid this in the past because their house was too small. But now that they had a new and larger home, it was assumed that the whole family, including aunts, uncles, and cousins, would meet at Raquel's house for Christmas. Raquel did not have a good relationship with her in-laws. Her mother-in-law had always been very picky about food and was easily offended if Raquel and her husband did not buy her the right gift. The mother-in-law had been known to be judgmental and a gossip. Because of this, Raquel and her husband had decided to keep Raquel's illness a secret. Raquel was afraid that her mother-in-law would somehow find out that she had bipolar disorder when she visited for Christmas and would confront her in front of the whole family. Raquel convinced herself that her only hope was to put together such a perfect celebration that there would be no need to be nervous and no reason to question her sanity.

To reduce catastrophic thinking you have to get the situation into perspective and plan ahead for whatever happens. Getting something into perspective means seeing it for what it is, not magnifying, not jumping to conclusions, and not making inaccurate assumptions. If you know which outcome is most likely to occur, you can plan ahead for it. If you control the outcome, it may not turn out as bad as you think, or at least if you know with certainty that a situation is not going to turn out well, you can plan ahead to deal with the consequences. To control catastrophizing, work through the sequence of steps on Worksheet 8.12.

Personalization

If you know that you have a tendency to take things personally when depressed or irritable, take that fact into consideration before you overreact. Here is an example of what Amanda has learned say to herself to help her cope when it seems like she is being ignored at work.

> *It feels like she ignored me on purpose, but I know that I'm kind of sensitive about that. Maybe she didn't see me, or maybe she had something else on her mind.*

By taking your sensitivity into consideration, you open your mind to other explanations for events that are less personal than you originally thought. If you can consider all possibilities, you're in a better position to figure out the conclusion that is most likely to be true. If you have considered alternative explanations for your experience and you're still uncertain whether or not to take something personally, ask someone else's opinion or ask the person who upset you. Be sure the topic is worth discussing. **Here are some questions to consider when you catch yourself taking things personally:**

- *Is it really about me?*
- *Could there be another explanation?*
- *Is it possible that it has nothing to do with me?*
- *Is it about the other person?*
- *Is it important enough to worry about?*
- *Is it important enough to discuss?*
- *Am I just sensitive because I'm not feeling my best?*

How to Decatastrophize Your Thoughts

1. If you think it's possible that you're catastrophizing about something, write down what you imagine will happen. It helps if you can picture the situation in your mind.

2. Ask yourself how likely it is that the catastrophe you imagined will occur. Is it a 100% certainty? Is there a 50% chance? Pick a number based on what you know to be true, not just what you fear.

   It is _____% likely that the catastrophe I fear will actually happen.

3. Are there other outcomes, besides the one you imagined, that might be just as likely to occur? If so, what are the other possible options? Make a list.

   a.

   b.

   c.

   d.

   e.

   f.

4. Cross off the list the possibilities that are the least likely to occur. This might include your original fear.

5. Of the items remaining, choose the mostly likely outcome.

   The most likely outcome of this situation is _____

   _____

   _____

   _____

6. Is there anything you can do to make things turn out better? Is there anything others can do for you that would make the situation turn out better? If so, what are the possibilities?

7. If you are right and the situation turns out to be catastrophic, how will you cope? How can you prepare yourself to deal with the aftermath?

Raquel's Worksheet 8.12

1. If you think it's possible that you're catastrophizing about something, write down what you imagine will happen. It helps if you can picture the situation in your mind.

    My mother-in-law will find out that I have bipolar disorder while she is visiting me, either by seeing my medication or because I am so uptight that I start acting hyper. My husband and kids might also give it away. She will get upset about it and confront me in front of others. I will probably cry and not be able to handle it. I will be humiliated, and everyone else will be so uncomfortable that they'll leave early.

2. Ask yourself how likely it is that the catastrophe you imagined will occur. Is it a 100% certainty? Is there a 50% chance? Pick a number based on what you know to be true, not just what you fear.

    It is 30 % likely that the catastrophe I fear will actually happen.

3. Are there other outcomes, besides the one you imagined, that might be just as likely to occur? If so, what are the other possible options? Make a list.

    a. *She will be too caught up in the celebration to notice.*
    b. *If she does notice, she won't say anything.*
    c. *The event will go smoothly. I won't get nervous or hyper.*
    d. *I will get hyper, but she'll think it's normal for me.*
    e. *She already knows I have bipolar disorder and will say nothing.*
    f. *My husband will deal with her before she says anything to the other relatives.*

4. Cross off the list the possibilities that are the least likely to occur. This might include your original fear.

    a. *~~She will be too caught up in the celebration to notice.~~*
    b. *If she does notice, she won't say anything.*
    c. *The event will go smoothly. I won't get nervous or hyper.*
    d. *~~I will get hyper, but she'll think it's normal for me.~~*
    e. *~~She already knows I have bipolar disorder and will say nothing.~~*
    f. *My husband will deal with her before she says anything to the other relatives.*

5. Of the items remaining, choose the mostly likely outcome.

    The most likely outcome of this situation is I will be nervous, but not hyper. If she thinks something is wrong, she will ask my husband and he will handle it for me.

Raquel's Worksheet 8.12 *(cont.)*

6. Is there anything you can do to make things turn out better? Is there anything others can do for you that would make the situation turn out better? If so, what are the possibilities?

   If I'm prepared before everyone arrives, it will go better.

   I can make sure there is time for a short rest before everyone arrives, rather than scrambling until the last minute.

   I can take a Xanax if I feel that my anxiety is getting out of control.

   I can ask my husband to run interference with his mother if it looks like she is putting me on the spot.

   I can stop worrying about what my mother-in-law thinks and focus more on pleasing my children and my husband.

7. If you are right and the situation turns out to be catastrophic, how will you cope? How can you prepare yourself to deal with the aftermath?

   If my mother-in-law starts to confront me, my husband will stop her. If he can't stop her, I will try to stay calm and address her concerns with a brief answer. I will offer to talk to her about my problems after the party is over. I'm sure she would agree to that. I will talk to my husband ahead of time about what to tell her and what not to tell her. I will schedule an appointment with my therapist for after Christmas just in case things do not go well.

When Tommy overreacted to his mother's question about his taking medicine, his girlfriend helped him pose these questions to himself.

- **Is it really about me?** *Yes. It's about me and my medication.*

- **Could there be another explanation?** *Maybe I was looking wigged out. Maybe my mom was just worried about me.*

- **Is it possible that it has nothing to do with me?** *No, it was about me and my medicine, not anyone else's problem.*

- **Is it about the other person?** *My mom can't stay out of my life. She treats me like her baby still. She doesn't trust me to take care of myself. She has always been like that.*

- **Is it important enough to worry about?** *Probably not.*

- **Is it important enough to discuss?** *Maybe. I've told her to leave me alone about the medicine, but she doesn't listen to me. I can't talk to her on my own. Maybe I can get my dad to talk to her.*

- **Am I just sensitive because I'm not feeling my best?** *Possibly. I did kind of yell at her and storm out of there. I didn't used to be like that. I used to be able to deal with her better.*

CATCH IT!

Tunnel Vision

Seeing only the things that confirm your point of view and ignoring or disregarding information to the contrary is tunnel vision. When Amanda is depressed, she is convinced that she's a loser. She remembers the mistakes she has made, the decisions she regrets, and the goals that she never met. Focusing attention on the things that confirm your view is part of tunnel vision. This is Amanda's list of evidence that she is a loser:

- *Didn't finish college.*
- *Got married too young.*
- *Have too much debt.*
- *Married the wrong guy.*

To make her argument more convincing, Amanda has to ignore any information to the contrary. That means she has to overlook, forget, or refuse to acknowledge evidence that she is not a loser. Ignoring contrary evidence is the second aspect of tunnel vision. Here is a partial list of Amanda's evidence against the idea that she is a loser:

- *Finished a 2-year certificate program as a practical nurse and have been working in a hospital for several years.*
- *Got my husband to quit drinking and to hold a job.*
- *Started my church's child ministry program.*
- *Have a new car.*
- *People like me and respect me.*

Tunnel vision in mania is similar. When people are hypomanic or manic, they may see evidence that confirms their view and ignore evidence against their view. If their mood is euphoric, they will see evidence to confirm an overly positive idea and ignore negative input from others.

> Hypomanic Husband: *I have the greatest idea. . . .*
>
> Wife: *That is the dumbest thing I have ever heard. Are you sure you're taking your medication?*
>
> Hypomanic Husband: *You just have no imagination. You're holding me back. I could really be something.*

If a person's mood is irritable as an episode of mania starts, he or she will see things that confirm a negative view and ignore facts that don't fit the mind set he or she is in.

Raquel's brother, Stan, for example, gets paranoid when he is having a manic episode. He thinks people at work are against him. What Stan does not see is that when he is paranoid and fearful he acts differently toward people at work. His suspiciousness shows. He is guarded, communicates less with others, and accuses them of touching things on this desk, being mean to him, or failing to keep him informed. When Stan is like this, people tend to stay away from him. He is unpleasant, and the change from his usual jovial self is confusing. No one knows that he has bipolar disorder, although they suspect that something is wrong with him. Their changes in behavior toward Stan confirm his paranoia.

The part that Stan forgets, does not see, or ignores is the evidence that people at work are considerate and respectful of him. He also forgets that when he is becoming manic he does not trust people.

| worksheet 8.13 | **Tunnel Vision** |

Examples of when tunnel vision distorted my thinking:

CONTROL IT!

How to Get Out of the Tunnel

The way out of tunnel vision is to force yourself to look at the big picture. When you're limiting yourself to looking at events that confirm a negative outlook, ask yourself or others if you're missing anything. Are you missing the situations in which

- Things have gone right?
- Problems have been solved effectively?
- People were kind to you?
- You received positive feedback?
- You were able to take action?

The same is true for overly positive tunnel vision when you're trying to convince yourself or others that everything is fine, that all things will work out, or that there's nothing to worry about. Are you missing:

- Times you were wrong?
- Mistakes in judgment that caused you problems?
- Periods when too much optimism clouded your thinking?
- Manic symptoms or signs that you are getting manic?
- The risks involved in your choices?

The overall goal is to examine all available information before you draw a conclusion. Look at the good news and the bad news, the evidence that your idea is right and that it is wrong, and then decide what to think.

When Tommy is angry with his parents, he looks at them with tunnel vision. He thinks about how they insist that he has bipolar disorder and bug him every day to take medication. He remembers the times they put him in a hospital when he knew he could take care of himself. When he is in one of those states of mind, he can easily convince himself that his parents do not care about him. To get out of the bad mood that usually accompanies tunnel vision, Tommy has to force himself to look at the whole story and to recognize that when he is mad it is easy to blame his parents and assume they have bad intentions toward him. Using the questions presented above, Tommy considers evidence that his parents might care about him.

- *Things have gone right*: They have done things right for him more than they have wronged him throughout his life. They have provided him with an apartment and a car and have helped him with money when he was between jobs.
- *Problems have been solved effectively*: This did not seem to apply to his situation.
- *People were kind to you*: His parents are usually kind to him unless he gets in their faces and accuses them of not caring.
- *You received positive feedback*: They say that they care, and they seem to be willing to do whatever it takes to help him.
- *You were able to take action*: This one does not apply to his situation.
- *After looking at the big picture, try to draw a conclusion that takes in all the information you have*. Tommy concluded that his parents cared about him a great deal; they just didn't always know how to handle him and did not always give him what he thought he needed.

CATCH IT!

Absolutes

Absolutes are rigid views of self, others, or life that are overly harsh, perfectionistic, or uncompromising. Seeing yourself as either a success or a failure, seeing others as either good or bad, and believing that there is a right way or a wrong way to do most things are all examples of absolutes. There is no middle ground; everything is either black or white. These extreme views make it hard on you during periods of your life when you're not doing well and unable to perform at the high level you've come to expect of yourself. If your definition of success is too stringent and you cannot fully reach it, you might think you're a failure.

Absolute thinking can also include seeing others in black-and-white terms; either they are meeting your expectations or they have failed you. When this happens, you might feel disappointed or let down and show it in your behavior. This can create tension in your relationships with others.

Absolutes can take many forms. Three of the more common ones are described in the sections that follow. They are black-and-white thinking, labeling, and shoulds. As you read through each example, think of ways in which you might find yourself thinking in absolute terms. Challenge yourself to rethink your view and see the shades of gray between the black and white extremes.

> **Black-and-white thinking: Categorical view in absolute terms such as good or bad, success or failure.**

When you talk in black-and-white terms you make it sound like there is no in-between, no compromise. Although you logically know that there are shades of gray between the black and white extremes, you may find those compromises unacceptable. Listen to your own language when you speak or as you think and try to identify examples of black and white ideas like the ones in the examples provided. Try your hand at finding an in-between way to look at things and avoid the extremes.

In the following examples, Raquel, Amanda, and Paul are seeing themselves or their situations in absolute terms because they are upset. In those moments, they believe that their extremely negative views are a true reflection of what is going on. Their negative thoughts stir up a lot of negative emotions. When you think in absolute terms, it's easy to assume that there are only two choices, good and bad. Raquel, Amanda, and Paul think that their situations are completely bad, and they think they know how they are supposed to be instead—completely good. If they were able to see the shades of gray between the black and white extremes, they would probably realize that their situations are not as bad as they seem. Furthermore, if they could be honest with themselves, they would see that wanting their situations to be perfect is not very realistic. Somewhere between perfect and terrible is where most people live. If they could aim for more realistic goals, between the black and white extremes, they would probably find that they are closer to a satisfactory level of performance than they originally thought.

Raquel comes home from a long and upsetting day at work and sees that her husband has left newspapers all over the living room, cups out on the counter, and his shoes in the middle of the floor. She thinks to herself, "This place is a dump."

Bad—How she sees it	In-between	Good—What she wants
The house is a complete dump.	House is not dirty, but is a little messy. Enough laundry is done to get us through the week.	The house is perfect. All laundry caught up. Everything put away. No dust.

When Amanda is feeling tired or stressed and is having a bad day at work, she tells herself that she hates her job.

Bad—How she sees it	In-between	Good—What she wants
This is the worst job in the world.	The job is OK. People are friendly. The tasks are interesting at times.	This is the job of my dreams. Fulfilling, profitable, great location, excellent benefits.

Paul gets a term paper back from his professor with a grade of C+ and is completely knocked off his feet. He thought that he deserved an A on it. He criticizes himself for doing badly.

Bad—How he sees it	In-between	Good—What he wants
I am a total failure in school.	I had to go to junior college for three years before transferring to university. No financial aid, but tuition is cheap and I will graduate next year.	"A" average. High enough SAT scores to get into the best college. Awarded a scholarship.

Fill in a personal example of black-and-white thinking in Worksheet 8.14. If you cannot think of an example of your own, listen to people around you and write in an example of something you've heard.

worksheet 8.14 | **Black, White, and In-Between Thinking**

Bad—How you see it	In-between	Good—What you want

CONTROL IT!

How to Control Black-and-White Thinking

There are some simple steps for controlling black-and-white thinking. They will help you find the middle between the extremes.

• **Step 1: Become aware** of the words you use that sound like extremes, black or white, or just too strong or harsh, like "I have the worst job in the world."

• **Step 2:** Ask yourself if the term you are using is accurate. If not, modify your thought to **make it more accurate.** For example, "It's not the worst job, but there are several things I don't like about it."

• **Step 3:** If you are not able to modify the thought, **write down on a piece of paper what each extreme would really look like.** For example, what would the absolute worst job in the world look like and what would the absolute best job in the world look like?

Worst job	Best Job
Pay is low.	*Pay higher than I really deserve.*
Conditions are harsh.	*Get to work at home in my pajamas.*
Schedule is bad.	*I can work when I want.*
People are mean.	*People adore me.*
What I do is illegal or immoral.	*Task is for the good of all mankind.*

• **Step 4: Ask yourself what the middle would look like.** What would a job be like if it were halfway between the best and the worst? Put yourself on the continuum between the extremes. Do you really have the worst job in the world?

• **Step 5: What are you going to do about it?** It's one thing to complain; it's quite another to fix the problem. If you are not pleased with yourself and your performance or aspects of your life are too close to the negative end of the black-and-white continuum, it's time to make some changes. Make a plan for moving your situation closer your goal.

CATCH IT!

> **Labeling: Using global critical labels for self or others such as stupid or lazy rather than looking at specific situations or behaviors.**

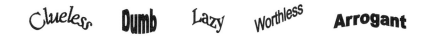

When someone cuts you off in traffic, behaves rudely, or says something on television that you strongly disagree with, it is not uncommon to call the person a name like *jerk* or *idiot* or *loser*. Sometimes we do it out loud and sometimes we do it in our heads. When we use negative labels for people we know, it is usually accompanied by negative feelings. In those moments, the label defines how we feel about the person, so it's easy to act as if the label were accurate. If you say that a person is irresponsible, you won't give them responsibilities. If you say a person is worthless, you will not treat the person with respect. Because labels are usually too extreme, the person who receives one will usually be offended by it. You would be too if the label were directed at you. Hurt feelings can interfere with good communication, cause conflict, and create or worsen tension in a relationship. Relationship stress can worsen symptoms of depression or mania.

When you're upset, it's not unusual to use harsh labels on yourself. Words like *stupid, pathetic,* or *lazy* don't fully describe what has happened, don't help you understand yourself better, and don't give you any direction for improvement. They just make you feel bad and reinforce your low self-esteem. If you automatically call yourself names like *stupid* when things go wrong, chances are you've made a habit of it. Using labels against yourself serves no good purpose. It only drags you down further and potentially worsens depression or keeps it from improving. In addition, thinking of yourself as stupid or lazy or pathetic keeps you from doing positive things in life. You hear the label and believe it's accurate, so you become convinced that you can't be any different. Labels can keep you from taking chances that would improve your life, making changes that are needed, and making progress toward feeling better or toward accomplishing your goals. The table on the following page provides some examples of how labels can cause you problems.

The Problem with Emotional Labels

Labels are a problem because they can:	For example, if I call myself a complete fool for trusting someone who later hurt me, it:
Make you feel bad.	*Makes me feel bad about myself.*
Be an exaggeration of the truth.	*Is not exactly accurate because I usually make good decisions about people.*
Be an incomplete or inaccurate description of the upsetting event.	*Wasn't just me being a fool. He was dishonest about his feelings.*
Be used as weapons against others.	*Only hurts me to say that I'm a fool. He is the one who should be hurting.*
Interfere with figuring out how to change.	*Doesn't help me figure out how to be more cautious in the future.*

CONTROL IT!

Alternatives to Labeling

Rather than applying a label to yourself or others, **try to describe the situation more fully.** Identify the specific actions or events that bothered you. Rather than saying to yourself "I'm lazy," try describing the situation more specifically, like "I didn't clean the kitchen today like I told myself I would and I am upset about that."

Once you have clearly described the problem, **make a plan for addressing it.** Be sure the plan is something realistic and under your control. For example, a plan for the kitchen might be "I'm going to start cleaning as soon as I get home today or as soon as I wake up in the morning."

When the label applies to someone else, try to describe the behavior that bothered you and ask yourself if there is anything you need to do about it or can do about it. If the answer is yes, take action. If the answer is no, let the event go and focus your attention on something more important to you or something you can control.

Instead of using emotional labels:

1. Describe the specific behavior that bothered you.
2. Make a plan for addressing this behavior.
3. If the label applies to someone else, describe the behavior that led you to use a label.
4. Is there anything you can do about the other person's behavior?
5. If yes, take action to solve the problem.
6. If no, drop the issue. Focus your attention on something you can control.

When Raquel thought about her mother-in-law, the label *control freak* came to mind. Others have used the same label and have complained about the mother-in-law's pickiness. In preparation for her mother-in-law's visit, Raquel decided to try to figure out what she could do about it. Since *control freak* is an emotional label, she tried the exercise for labeling.

- **If the label applies to someone else, describe the behavior that led you to use a label.** *My mother-in-law wants to tell everyone where they should sit at the dinner table even when it is not her house.*
- **Is there anything you can do about the other person's behavior?** *I can tell her that at my house I get to decide where everyone will sit. I can put out name cards at each place setting before my mother-in-law arrives for dinner.*
- **If yes, take action to solve the problem.** *I will put the name cards out and see how she reacts.*
- **If no, drop the issue. Focus your attention on something you can control.** *If she insists on having her way, I will let it go. It is not worth the risk of creating disagreement at a family dinner.*

CATCH IT!

> *Shoulds: Unbending rules about how you think people should act or think or how you think things in the world should be.*

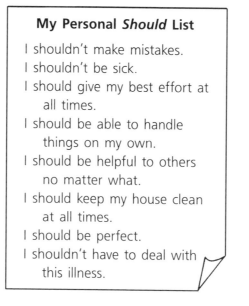

My Personal *Should* List

I shouldn't make mistakes.
I shouldn't be sick.
I should give my best effort at all times.
I should be able to handle things on my own.
I should be helpful to others no matter what.
I should keep my house clean at all times.
I should be perfect.
I shouldn't have to deal with this illness.

Most people have *should* lists but may not be fully aware of it. *Should*s are unwritten rules that you learn early in life, usually from your family. They are sometimes called *values* or *beliefs*. The problem is that *should*s are absolute and unbending, and when you cannot live up to them you feel bad about yourself. These rules could be appropriate in the perfect world where we are able to function at our best at all times, no obstacles interfere with our goals, people act the way we expect, and everything runs smoothly. Few, if any, people live in that kind of world. And if you have bipolar disorder, you cannot guarantee that things will always go the right way. The illness causes symptoms that interfere with your ability to function at your best. Other people will behave in ways that cause you stress and make you feel worse, and things do not always turn out the way they should. That's the dilemma for someone who has bipolar disorder. On the one hand you think your *should* list represents rules you have to live by despite having an illness. On the other hand, you can't always make things turn out the way you think they should be either because you do not have control over all aspects of life or because you are not always able to function as well as you'd like. This causes great frustration, aggravation, and guilt.

To add to the stress, most of us have a *should* list for other people in our lives, like the one below, and when those people do not perform in the way they are expected to, we feel angry, disappointed, and hopeless.

Should List for Others

Other people should:

Be kind.
Be courteous.
Be thoughtful.
Be on time.
Be patient.
Be willing to help.
Be available.
Be responsible.

CONTROL IT!

Changing *Should*s to *Want*s

If you feel disappointed in yourself or others because your expectations are not being met, it is probably time to change your rigid expectations to something with more flexibility. Rather than stating the *should* as a rule, soften it by restating it as a preference. The table below provides some examples of how you can change your *should*s into preferences and plans. If you change your way of thinking about how things should be and focus more on what you prefer, many opportunities for change can emerge. For example, instead of stating, "I shouldn't make mistakes," you can restate it as "I don't like to make mistakes, so I'll try to slow down, think things through, and make better decisions." Restating *should*s in less rigid terms gives you a goal to work toward rather than a rule you punish yourself for breaking.

Changing Shoulds

*Should*s	Preferences and plans
I shouldn't be sick.	I wish I didn't have this illness. I will do what I can to keep it from interfering with my life.
I should give my best effort at all times.	I'm not always able to give my best, but I want to do the best I can as often as possible.
I should be able to handle things on my own.	I would rather not be a burden to others. I will ask my family for help if I really need it.
I should not have bipolar disorder.	No one should have this illness. I would rather have perfect health. I will do my part to feel better.
I should be helpful to others no matter what.	I like helping others but do not always have the energy. I will help when I can.
I should keep my house clean at all times.	I love having a clean house, but it is not the end of the world if I can't keep it that way. I will try to keep it as clean as possible and not be upset with myself when I can't.
I should be perfect.	No one is perfect. I want to try to do the best I can in the areas that are most important to me.
I shouldn't have to deal with this illness.	I would prefer not to deal with it, but I don't have that choice. I will try to control it so it does not dominate my life.

Create your personal list of *should*s on Worksheet 8.15 and try to rephrase them as preferences that are less absolute or black and white.

➡️ *What's Next?*

You are now well on your way in learning to catch and correct your thinking errors. Thinking more clearly when you are depressed or manic will reduce the intensity of your mood swings. When your emotions and thinking errors are controlling your behavior, you will make mistakes, handle things badly, offend others, and cope poorly with problems. When you catch, control, and correct your errors in logic, these things are less likely to happen.

In the next chapter you will learn several other strategies for analyzing your reactions to upsetting events and correcting your distortions in thinking. These methods will help you reduce the cognitive and emotional symptoms of depression and mania.

| worksheet 8.15 | **Changing *Should*s** |

My *should*s	My preferences and plans

chapter nine

Controlling Emotional Thoughts

In this chapter you will:

✓ Be introduced to thought records.
✓ Learn how to evaluate the accuracy of your negative and manic thoughts.
✓ Counter thoughts of suicide by exploring reasons to live and reasons to have hope.

Thought Records

The Thought Record (Worksheet 9.1) is a tool to help you through the **triple-C method** of **catching** your distorted thoughts, **controlling** them so they do not negatively affect your actions, and **correcting** them so that you think more logically and rationally. Thought records provide a structure for listing thoughts that come to mind when you are troubled or distressed or when your emotions or symptoms may be influencing by your thinking. Advantages of using a thought record include the following:

- It is easier to write down your thoughts before trying to analyze or change them instead of trying to do it all in your head.
- You can have many thoughts at one time, all of which are important. Writing them out allows you to work on one at a time.
- Seeing your thoughts on paper can help you quickly identify errors in logic. It's easy to believe negative thoughts are true until you see them in writing.
- Negative thoughts tend to recur. So if you want to remember how you worked through a negative thought, keeping a thought record means you don't have to rely on your memory.
- If you want to share your work with your doctor or therapist, it is easier to provide the thought record than to try to recall an upsetting event and the thoughts and feelings you had at the time.

| **Thought Record**

Event What triggered your thoughts and feelings?	**Thoughts** Write down all the thoughts that popped into your mind when the event occurred. Put one thought in each box below.	**Feelings** What feelings were experienced? Include emotions and physical sensations.	**Thinking error** Can you identify any thinking errors?

Paul's Worksheet 9.1

Event	Thoughts	Feelings	Thinking error
Girlfriend did not return phone call.	She must be mad at me. She doesn't want to talk to me.	Sadness	Mind reading
	It's my fault for not returning her call right away last time.	Guilt	Personalizing
	I'm such a lousy boyfriend.	Guilt	Labeling
	I bet she's going to dump me.	Grief	Fortune telling

In this case Paul did not actually know why the girlfriend did not return his phone call, so he let his imagination fill in the blanks. When he saw his worries written on the thought record, he could not help noticing that each fell into one of the thinking error categories. This told him that he was probably letting his emotions take control of his thoughts. He followed the advice from Chapter 8 about jumping to conclusions and got more information by calling his girlfriend again.

Evaluating Your Thoughts

The immediate thoughts you have in response to an event might be overly negative or overly positive. Sometimes these will be distortions and sometimes these thoughts will be accurate. If you're not certain whether your thoughts are true or false, you will need to put them to a test. Below and on the next page are some ways to test your thoughts for accuracy.

Ways to Evaluate the Accuracy of Your Thoughts

1. Look back through your examples of **thinking errors** from the last chapter to see if your thoughts fall under one of those categories.

2. **Ask people** for their opinions. Do they see things the same way? Do they think you are being overly positive or overly negative?

3. Use Worksheet 9.2 (Evaluating Your Thoughts) to **write down all the evidence** you have that your thought is true. Write down all the evidence you have that your idea is false. Compare the evidence.

4. Make yourself **consider other possible explanations** for the events that upset you or aroused your emotions. Is it possible that you jumped to the first conclusion that came to mind? Remember that your first thoughts are not always your most accurate thoughts. They are just your first thoughts.

5. Ask yourself **what you would tell another person** who was in the same situation. Pretend you're giving feedback to another person. Write it down and follow your own suggestions.

---

worksheet 9.2 | **Evaluating Your Thoughts**

My thought is: _____

What evidence do I have that my thought is true?	What evidence do I have that my thought is not true?	What would someone else say in this situation? What is another explanation?	My conclusions and my plan for what to do next

Amanda provides a good example of how to think through an upsetting situation by testing out the validity of some negative thoughts that were stirred up by an upsetting event. She received a notice in the mail that it was time for her to renew her nursing license. The new application had a place for reporting whether or not she had been treated or is being treated for a mental illness. This was a new part of the application since the last time she had renewed her license. No one in nursing knew that Amanda had bipolar disorder, and she did not want to have to tell anyone. She was very upset about the implications of this new rule. She wrote down her immediate thoughts on the thought record to try to get her bearings on the situation.

All of Amanda's thoughts fall into the category of jumping to conclusions. She noticed this but was still not convinced that the thoughts were false. What fueled her fears was mistrust of her boss, of her coworkers, and of the state nursing board. Even

Amanda's Worksheet 9.1

Event	Thoughts	Feelings	Thinking error
Finding out that I would have to report that I had bipolar disorder to the nursing board	This is horrible. They are not going to renew my license. I will be out of work. We are not going to be able to pay our bills.	Fear	Catastrophizing
	The nursing board is going to have to tell my employer, and everyone at work will know that I have bipolar disorder.	Anger Frustration	Fortune telling
	When my boss finds out, she is going to think that I can't take care of patients. She will watch me like a hawk and find a reason to fire me.	Anger Fear	Mind reading
	My boss will tell others, and I will be completely humiliated.	Embarrassment	Fortune telling

when Amanda is not upset, she thinks that her boss, coworkers, and the nurses on the state board try to appear supportive but are capable of stabbing her in the back. Her instinct was to lie on her application or to refuse to complete that item even though both of those options could have negative consequences. Her immediate course of action was to avoid sending in her renewal application for as long as possible.

After completing the thought record and deciding which thinking errors she might have made, Amanda picked the one that bothered her most and tried to analyze it.

Amanda's Worksheet 9.2

My thought is: They are not going to renew my license. I will be out of work. We are not going to be able to pay our bills.			
What evidence do I have that my thought is true?	What evidence do I have that my thought is not true?	What would someone else say in this situation? What is another explanation?	My conclusions and my plan for what to do next
If you do not have a license, you cannot practice nursing in a hospital. Licenses are checked every year. There has been a trend in recent years of reprimanding nurses with substance abuse problems. Those who have lost their licenses are listed in the state board bulletin each year. Many nurses will not take medication for depression because they are afraid of losing their jobs.	The application does not say that I will lose my license. I haven't heard of anyone other than those with substance abuse problems losing their licenses. It would be discrimination to take away your license just because you've been in treatment. There are laws against that. My husband says that I can't lose my license over this.	Someone else would say that I won't know unless I ask. My husband says it's just a bureaucratic maneuver. The nursing board is not going to put itself at risk of getting sued by a bunch of nurses. They can't violate your privacy by telling your boss about your illness.	Find a way to anonymously ask about the rules. Find out what the consequences would be if I lied about my illness. Find out if and how the board will check on the truthfulness of answers to questions about mental illness. If I find out that the board is going to take action on my license, hire a lawyer to help me with this. Renew my application on time. Don't delay it and draw attention to my case.

When you look at evidence for and against a thought, you have to take into consideration the importance of each piece of evidence before you draw any conclusions. It's possible that one column will have a lot more evidence than the other. This does not necessarily mean that the column with more items is more valid. You have to take into consideration how much each item influences your belief in the idea you're testing.

Amanda knows that what makes her fear most believable is that other nurses have said they won't take medications or see a counselor when they need one because they're afraid of losing their jobs. On the opposite side of the argument, what makes her worry less is that she trusts her husband's judgment. Ultimately, she will have to get more information about this new reporting rule before she will feel any relief.

Amanda made a plan to get as much information as she could before she turned in her renewal application. She will start with a nurse she knows at a different hospital. Sally is older than Amanda and also has bipolar disorder. Sally keeps up on the state board rules and may be able to address Amanda's concerns. If she doesn't know, Sally will know who to ask without getting into trouble.

Amanda considered quitting her job and letting her license expire, but decided it would be better to be let go than to leave voluntarily. She did not want to make it easy for them to discriminate against her.

Amanda analyzed each of her worries on the Thought Record using the methods described. Working through her thoughts in a systematic way did not take away all of Amanda's anxiety or anger, but it did help her calm down enough to come up with a reasonable plan for dealing with her problem.

Tommy is learning to use Thought Records to cope with the ideas he gets when he is becoming manic. The last few times he got manic, he had the urge to take a trip. One time he got in his car and drove until he ran out of gas. He had forgotten his wallet, so he had to call his mom to come bring him gasoline. She refused to let him drive his car, so he had to go home with her. Another time, he bought a round-trip ticket to Hawaii on a credit card his father had given him to use for school expenses. He left without telling anyone where he was going. He hung out at the beach for a few days but did not have any fun. When he came back his parents were furious and canceled his credit card. Tommy practiced with his therapist how to analyze his urges to travel before he goes on the road.

When the urge to leave town hits him, Tommy always gets the idea that he has to follow his instinct or he'll go crazy. Every minute he waits feels like an eternity. He also tends to have the idea that everything will turn out fine if he goes. There will be no negative consequences, only relief from the pressure he feels. During a therapy visit, when the urge to travel was only mild, Tommy and his therapist worked through the steps to analyze these thoughts.

Tommy's Worksheet 9.1

Event	Thoughts	Feelings	Thinking error
Got the urge to go to Hawaii.	I want to go to Hawaii this weekend. I need to get away from the cold weather. It's a good idea.	Excited	No
	I will feel better if I go to Hawaii.	Excited	Could be fortune telling in a good way
	I don't care about the money. I deserve a break.	Confident	Personalization
	If I don't get out of town, I'm going to go crazy.	Stressed	Catastrophizing

Tommy's Worksheet 9.2

My thought is: If I don't get out of town, I'm going to go crazy.			
What evidence do I have that my thought is true?	What evidence do I have that my thought is not true?	What would someone else say in this situation? What is another explanation?	My conclusions and my plan for what to do next
I can feel myself getting more uptight each day. I can't stand being in my apartment every day. I hate the cold weather. I always feel better when I'm at the beach.	No one actually goes crazy because they can't travel. I've felt this way before. The urge eventually goes away.	My mother would say that I'm manic again. My father would probably agree. It is the middle of the semester, and if I miss any more classes, I will probably fail them.	I will plan a trip to Hawaii during spring break if I still have the urge to go by then. I'll do other things to control my restless feelings. I will take the medication the doctor gave me and work out at the gym more often.

Tommy's Worksheet 9.2

My thought: *It's a good idea to go to Hawaii.*			
What evidence do I have that my thought is true?	What evidence do I have that my thought is not true?	What would someone else say in this situation? What is another explanation?	My conclusions and my plan for what to do next
I love the beach. I hate the cold weather at home. I can get a cheap fare for this weekend.	*I would have to miss my Friday class. I don't have the money to pay for a trip right now. My father is going to be mad when he gets the credit card bill.*	*My sister would say that no one likes cold weather, but you can't just take off in the middle of the semester. My brother would say it was stupid to go to Hawaii right now. My friend says the fares are cheap because no one is going there right now. There won't be any action. When I have taken off on trips like this before, things have turned out badly.*	*It's a dumb idea. I'm not going to Hawaii right now.*

After you've completed your thought record and thought analysis, go back and examine your original thoughts. Can you see how being objective changes your thoughts? What did you notice about the intensity of the emotions you originally felt? If your emotions are still pretty intense, try one of the other methods mentioned in this chapter and Chapter 8 for coping with your emotional thoughts.

Thoughts about Suicide

There may be times when thoughts about death or suicide seem reasonable or perhaps comforting. Severe depression can darken your thinking to such a degree that you might be able to convince yourself that dying is your only option. These are scary thoughts that often lead to hurtful acts against yourself in an attempt to take your own life.

Suicidal thoughts can take many forms. In their most severe form, you might hear voices instructing you to kill yourself. These are auditory hallucinations, triggered by the biological changes occurring in your brain when you are depressed. They are not your true thoughts. A milder form of suicidal thoughts might include vague ideas about dying or a desire to just run away or disappear. In the middle range, there might be thoughts that it would be OK with you if your death occurred, although you wouldn't necessarily do anything to bring it about. Some people wish they could fall asleep peacefully and not wake up.

Thoughts about death or suicide are usually the result of feeling hopeless about the future and helpless to make anything change. When you can't think of any other solutions to your problems and can see no reason to hold on, death may begin to seem like an acceptable option.

To have a chance to change your life for the better, you have to stick around long enough to learn something new. Try the exercise in Worksheet 9.3 to help you fight off thoughts about death and dying. List your reasons to live. Plan ahead for times when you might have doubts that life is worth living. List things you would want to remind yourself of when times are bad.

Paul went through a few serious bouts of depression and even tried to kill himself with an overdose of pills. He remembers working his way out of wanting to die by thinking of reasons to stick around. Here is his list.

Paul's Worksheet 9.3

Reasons I shouldn't leave:

There are things I wanted to do with my life.
I want to finish college and get a job.

People to live for:

My mom, my grandmother, my girlfriend, my best friend, my nieces, my brother

Things I would miss:

Hockey games, the Super Bowl, sausage pizza, sex

Experiences I have not yet had:

I want to buy a new car.
I want to see the Grand Canyon.
I want to learn to scuba dive.

Things that matter to me:

My family and my friends

Make a list of reasons to continue living. When you begin to have dark thoughts about life, look over the list to remind yourself of these reasons to hold on for another day.

Reasons I shouldn't leave:

People to live for:

Things I would miss:

Experiences I have not yet had:

Things that matter to me:

Reasons to Have Hope

When you feel depressed enough to have suicidal thoughts, you might think there is no other way to solve your problems. You may have temporarily lost confidence in your ability to pull out of the slump you're in. When others try to encourage you or express their confidence in your ability to get better, you might minimize it because it does not fit with your negative view at the time. There may be good reasons to be hopeful about the future, but the tunnel vision that clouds your thinking when you are severely depressed does not let you see them. Because of this, it's best to make your list of reasons to have hope at a time when you are feeling more confident and hopeful. When you're depressed, you can read the list to remind yourself that your outlook can be more positive and that part of you knows there are reasons to be hopeful.

On Worksheet 9.4, make a list of reasons that you believe there might be hope for your future. Here are some questions that might help you think of reasons to have hope.

- Are you doing anything now that might suggest there is hope for improvement? Are there things you could do?
- Are the problems that bring you down likely to be temporary? Will they resolve themselves with time?
- Why do other people believe there is hope for the future?
- Is it possible that you have not yet given it all your effort?
- Have you been through times like this before? Have things usually gotten better with time, effort, or patience?

Review your list from time to time and add new reasons you can think of to be hopeful. Keep the list where you will be able to find it when you start to doubt that life is worth living.

Caution!

- Fantasies about suicide can be very **seductive**. They can trick you into thinking that death will be better than life.
- Fantasies about suicide can give you **false comfort**. They can fool you into believing that death is the reasonable solution to your problems.
- Fantasies about suicide **delude you** into thinking that no one will mind. They allow you to conjure up fake images of everyone being better off without you. They do not allow you to see the grief and misery you will leave behind. They keep you from imagining the guilt that will plague your family and friends for not having saved you.
- Fantasies are not only dangerous for you; they **set a dangerous standard** for

Reasons for Hope

My reasons for hope:

Amanda's Worksheet 9.4

My reasons for hope:

I have a lot of people in my life who love me and help me through difficult times.

I have gotten depressed and lost hope before, but I have also gotten it back.

I am a strong person. If I can survive childbirth, I can survive this.

I always think this way when I'm depressed. It will pass.

I have a good doctor and a good therapist who will help me survive.

My kids are my reason for hope.

I just started on a new medication that the doctor thinks will pull me out of this.

I know there is more I can do to help myself.

others. Children who have a parent who has committed suicide are more likely to commit suicide themselves. Suicide can mean condemning those you love you to a similar fate.

Clinicians take even your vaguest thoughts of suicide seriously, and so should you. They know that a general notion that life may not be worth living or that you would like to go to sleep and never wake up can turn into an active plan to commit suicide. Sometimes clinicians, family members, and friends may seem to overreact when you make comments that suggest that death is on your mind. They overreact because they don't know how close you are to acting on these ideas. While you may take comfort in thoughts about death, they feel a sense of panic and responsibility for your well-being. They don't want to lose you even if in those moments you are not worried about losing them.

Do not wait until the last minute to ask for help. If you find that you have active thoughts about killing yourself or less specific ideas that death would be all right with you, tell someone about it. Tell a family member, call your doctor or therapist, or ask a member of the clergy for help. Do not trust yourself to set limits on your suicidal fantasies. Get help if you experience any of the following:

- Thoughts about suicide, including fantasies about how you might do it.
- Recurrent thoughts about death in general.
- Envy for people who are dead or who are dying.

- You find yourself giving away your possessions.
- You hear yourself saying good-bye to family members, friends, or pets.
- You begin to prepare people to live without you.
- You become aware of things in your environment that can help you commit suicide.
- You start to hoard your medication so you will have enough for an overdose.
- Warning labels look like prescriptions for suicide.

The goal of this workbook is to teach you ways to control your symptoms of depression and mania before they get to the point that suicide starts to be an attractive idea. If you use the exercises for monitoring your mood changes, be as consistent as you can with your medication, and learn the methods presented so far for controlling your symptoms, you can stop episodes of depression and mania from getting out of control.

What's Next?

You have learned many different methods for dealing with distorted thinking. You can use the Thought Records to catch emotional thoughts and reason through them using the methods covered in the last chapter and this one. Remember that the easiest way to catch distorted thoughts is to notice shifts in your mood. When you find yourself overly excited or upset, ask yourself what it is about the situation that is affecting your mood. Once you identify your thoughts, you can sort out logical thoughts from emotional thoughts.

Another way that your cognitions can cause you trouble is when your thought process gets bogged down, when concentration is poor, when thoughts are disorganized, and when it is hard for you to make decisions. The next chapter offers strategies for slowing, focusing, and structuring your thoughts so that you can concentrate better, make decisions, and solve problems. When you're able to organize your thoughts, you'll make better choices of action and handle life more effectively.

chapter ten

Reversing Mental Meltdown

In this chapter you will:

✓ Identify ways that your thinking becomes confused or disorganized.

✓ Learn the *slow it, focus it, structure it* method of coping with mental meltdown.

✓ Discover new ways to organize your thoughts and make decisions.

One of the more common complaints that people with bipolar disorder have is that their thinking gets slowed, confused, disorganized, cluttered, and unfocused. They can't make decisions, have trouble reading, don't know which thought to tend to first, have trouble conversing with others, and in general lack clarity in their thinking. These are called *cognitive processing problems*. They can be extremely frustrating and can keep you from accomplishing even the smallest goals, whether you are newly diagnosed or have had bipolar disorder for a while. Unfortunately, frustration, aggravation, and annoyance only make cognitive processing more difficult. The exercises in this chapter are intended to help you cope with mental meltdown. The following table provides some examples of the types of cognitive processing problems people have when they are depressed and when they are manic.

Coping with Mental Meltdown

The general strategy for coping with cognitive processing problems is to **first** slow down the process of thinking and decision making enough to be able to get a handle on it. **Second**, focus your attention on one idea at a time. **Third**, use a systematic method for making decisions or drawing conclusions.

Examples of Cognitive Processing Problems

Category of cognitive processing	Examples in depression	Examples in mania
Response to stimulation	Easily overwhelmed	Distracted easily Sounds seem louder Colors seem brighter
Speed in thinking	Slowed thinking Difficulty finding words or putting thoughts together	Racing thoughts More ideas or thoughts
Concentration	Cannot hold focus without mind wandering or going blank	Too many thoughts to process Distracted and lose train of thought
Organization	Cannot organize thoughts and problems efficiently enough to deal with them	Difficulty grasping and organizing thoughts
Decision making	Self-doubt interferes with decision making Problem solving is impaired	Cannot prioritize Judgment is impaired Cannot follow through with decisions

Slow it   by slowing the body and mind.
Focus it   on one idea at a time.
Structure it by using decision-making exercises.

Specific methods for slowing it, focusing it, and structuring it to gain control over mental meltdown are listed in the table below and will be described in this chapter. This chapter will show you how to use these strategies toward better organizing your thoughts and making decisions that are best for you.

Overview of Strategies to Cope with Mental Meltdown

Slow it	Focus it	Structure it
• Decrease stimulation —Internal thoughts —External noise • Relaxation exercises	• Pick one thing at a time • "A" list/"B" list • Prioritize with goal setting • Write it down and put it in front of you	• Problem solving • Advantages/disadvantages • Use Thought Records • Get feedback from others • Impose the 24-hour rule

Slow It

Thinking becomes muddled during depression and mania for many different reasons, but one common reason is that there is too much mental activity. Thoughts such as worries, ideas, ruminations, regrets, and self-criticism, as well as more random thoughts, are swimming around in your mind. If you're easily distracted, thoughts about things you hear, see, smell, or feel can also enter your mind even when you are not intentionally concentrating on them. When there is too much going on in your mind, it is hard to focus on any one thought long enough to see it through to its conclusions. This is not only the case during manic episodes; it can also happen during depression. Having too many things on your mind at once is stressful and confusing.

Slowing your mind can be difficult to achieve. Medications aimed at stabilizing mood and reducing anxiety can usually help. In addition, there are a few things that you can try. One strategy is to get away from distractions in your environment. When you remove yourself from overstimulating environments, your thoughts will be easier to control. This means turning off the television or radio, going to a quiet place in your home, or leaving places where there is too much noise or activity. It's hard to think when you're being bombarded with noise. Changing your environment can reduce stimulation and make it easier to think. When Amanda gets so mentally overwhelmed that she cannot think straight, she goes outside into her backyard and swings on her kids' swing or takes her dog for a walk around the block a few times just to get away from everything. Paul finds that if he puts his earphones on and listens to music in his room, he can escape the noise in his environment and in his head. Raquel likes to drive her car in silence with the radio off and the windows up. That seems to slow everything down for her.

Sometimes the noise in your environment is visual. That includes looking at unfinished tasks, clutter, piles of mail, dirty laundry, or other things that remind you of all the tasks you need to complete. This is a big problem for Amanda when her kids have their toys and schoolwork out, the table has a pile of mail on it, the kitchen is a mess after cooking dinner, and she is too tired to deal with it.

For ways to quiet your mind by reducing internal and external stimulation, return to Chapter 5. The methods described in the sections called "Reducing Environmental Stimulation" and "Reducing Internal Stimulation" will help you slow yourself down so you can sort through and organize your thoughts. When you are depressed and your mind is cluttered with regrets, worries, self-criticism, hopelessness, or suicidality, use the methods from Chapters 8 and 9 to change your thinking. Working through some of your thinking errors will also help you think more clearly.

Another strategy for slowing your thoughts enough to think them through is to slow down your body. Getting a good night's sleep is the obvious solution if sleep loss is interfering with your ability to concentrate and think. Methods for improving your sleep can be found in Chapter 5. If sleep loss is not the issue, your body may be wound up due to excess energy or muscle tension. Relaxing your body can help to relax your mind. Your doctor may have prescribed medications that relax you and calm your mind. If not, you can try relaxation exercises.

Relaxation Exercise

Find a comfortable and quiet place to sit or lie down. Take off your shoes, loosen your belt, take your hair out of your ponytail, or otherwise remove items that bind you too tightly. Keep a light on so you can read these instructions. **Take one deep breath** in through your nose and let it out through your mouth. As you do this, tell your body to let go of the tensions from head to toe. Continue to breathe normally and focus on releasing tensions from specific parts of your body. Let's **begin with your face.** Focus on relaxing your forehead. Smooth out any wrinkles, make your eyebrows relax, and think of tension dripping off your forehead and away from your body the way that sweat might drip off your forehead. Take a moment to loosen your forehead before going on.

When you're ready, turn your focus to your jaw and loosen it as much as you can. Let your teeth part, relax your jaw, releasing any tension you hold there. Loosen your jaw by letting your teeth part just a little. Release any tension you hold in your lips. Make sure your forehead stays relaxed and your jaw loose.

While keeping your eyes open enough to be able to read, try to relax your eyes. Feel tension leaving your face, falling away from your forehead, away from your eyes, and being released from your jaw. Your face is smoother, calmer, and more relaxed. Keep your face loose while you turn your attention to your shoulders and neck.

To begin to relax your **shoulders and neck,** let your shoulders drop and let your arms drop to your sides. Let the tension flow down your neck, down your shoulders, and away from your body. Picture your shoulder muscle being tight like a wet dishrag that you are wringing. Let your shoulders loosen just as you untwist the dishrag and shake it loose. Let the tension leave your neck and shoulders as you relax.

Let your attention go back to your face, search out any tightness you may have left there, and release it once again.

Next, it's time for allow your **arms** to relax. Starting at the top of your shoulders, allow the tension to leave those muscles. Feel your arms relax as you let them fall to your side. Relax your hands, let your fingers spread apart, and imagine tension flowing away from your body, down your arms, off your fingertips, and away from your body. Let your tensions melt away and drip off your fingertips and onto the floor like ice melting slowly.

Once again, focus on any remaining tension in your shoulders, allowing them to loosen further. Let relaxation flow through your face and neck, down your arms, and into your hands and fingers.

Now it's time to relax your **chest and stomach**. Continue to breathe normally, but as you exhale, focus on letting tension leave your body just as the air leaves your lungs. Feel relaxation spreading through your chest and stomach as you exhale. Take as long as you need to exhale away the tensions and breathe a sense of relaxation into your body.

Focus now on your stomach and allow it to relax. Release your stomach muscles, allowing them to loosen and feel more comfortable. Feel your body become more relaxed from your head to your shoulders, to your chest and throughout your stomach. Search out any tensions that remain and let them go free.

Now turn your attention to your **legs**. Uncross your legs or ankles if you have them crossed. Let the muscles relax throughout your legs and feet and all the way down to your toes. Loosen your toes, relax your ankles, and let your legs lie comfortably and relaxed. Imagine tension flowing down your legs, off your feet, and onto the floor.

Now **count from one to ten**, but as you say each number to yourself, try to relax just a little bit more. Let yourself focus on each group of muscles from head to toe, and when you find tension remaining, allow it to flow away from your body. **One**, focus on your face, letting go of any tension you find. **Two**, continue to let your shoulders drop and feel the tension flowing away from your neck and shoulders. **Three**, search your arms and hands and fingers. Allow them to continue to relax. **Four**, exhale, breathing out any remaining tensions in your chest. **Five**, loosen your stomach just a little bit more. **Six**, relax your right leg just a little bit more. Let it lie comfortably and loosely. **Seven**, turn your attention to your left leg. Allow it to loosen just a little bit more. **Eight**, once again scan your body from head to toe, find any remaining tensions in your muscles, and allow them to flow away from your body. **Nine**, as you exhale, notice that you're breathing more slowly and comfortably as you've allowed your body to slow down, to release the strains of the day, and to relax. **Ten**, enjoy the moment.

Memorize this feeling of relaxation. Notice how it is different from when you started this exercise. Tell your muscles to remember the sensation of relaxation so that you can go there again when you need to. Notice that your thoughts have slowed down. They are now easier to catch, and you can focus on the things that are most important to you at this moment. When you're ready, allow yourself to pick a goal or a thought that needs your attention. Focus your energy on that single idea and see it to its conclusion.

The 24-Hour Rule

Another strategy for slowing things down to give yourself a chance to think is to impose the 24-hour rule. This simply means holding off on making decisions or taking action for 24 hours when your plan involves doing something that you would not normally do, that others would object to, or that may involve some risks. This rule is based on the idea that if something is a good idea today, it will be a good idea tomorrow. In the meantime, use the other methods in this workbook to sort through your thoughts so that when you make a decision to act, it will not be something you later regret. If 24 hours is not enough time, make it a 48-hour rule. Tommy uses the 24-hour rule before he gives in to his urge to travel. Raquel uses the 24-hour rule when she gets the urge to overspend at the mall. Amanda uses the 24-hour rule before scolding her husband. She figures if an issue is worth risking marital conflict over, it will still be important the next day. If she gives herself 24 hours to cool off, she is more likely to handle the situation with tact instead of biting her husband's head off.

Focus It

The general rule of thumb for helping your mind focus is to work on one idea or task at a time. This is difficult to do if you have racing thoughts. That's why you have to slow your thought process with the methods described in the preceding section and in Chapter 5 before you take on a problem or big decision. Once you are able to slow down enough to choose a thought to work through, you must choose only one thing at a time. The goal-setting exercise and the "A" list/"B" list exercise you learned in Chapter 5 will help you narrow your focus. Once you've chosen the problem, idea, or decision to focus on, **write it down on a piece of paper and place it in front of you**. This is a simple exercise but can really help you stay on track. Tommy figures out which homework assignment he is going to work on first, gathers the materials he needs in front of him, and puts everything else away. This keeps his mind from wandering to different assignments from different classes.

You will be less likely to let your mind wander off to other topics if you keep your eye on the one you've chosen to work on. Make yourself finish whatever needs to be done on one problem before you go on to the next one. It's very easy to think of many other problems when you're working on one. If you can focus and take one thing off your mental "to do" list at a time, your mind will be less cluttered with stressful thoughts. Overall, you'll feel better.

If you catch your mind wandering to other topics as Raquel does, just tell yourself to go back and finish what you started. Raquel worries that if she does not take care of things as she thinks of them, she will forget to do them. She controls the urge to pursue tasks as they come to mind by writing herself a brief note about a new idea and going back to her original task. If it's written down, she will not forget to do it.

Paul does a similar thing when he works at his desk by making a note on a marker board he has on the wall. He put a smaller marker board in his kitchen for the same purpose. When he writes things down, he can keep his focus on one task at a time and go back to the others on the board when he finishes.

Structure It

The strategy you choose for structuring your thoughts will depend on the action that is needed. The table below summarizes the kinds of thoughts you might need to structure and the strategies that may be most helpful to you.

Problem Solving

• **Step 1: Define the problem.** The most difficult part of solving problems is clearly describing the nature of the problem. While difficult, it's an essential step. If you can clearly see the problem, you can solve it or cope with it. Using vague or general terms that do not fully describe what is happening will not lead you to a solution. Some examples of vague and clear definitions of problems are provided in the table on the facing page.

Ways to Cope with Mental Meltdown

Type of mental meltdown	*Strategy*
If you're having a difficulty or problem that needs to be resolved . . .	Use the problem-solving exercise described in the next section.
If you're having trouble making a decision about something important to you . . .	Skip ahead to the decision-making section of this chapter.
If you need to sort through upsetting or emotional thoughts . . .	Go back to Chapter 9 and use the Thought Records and the methods for evaluating your thinking.
If you're having trouble organizing your thoughts well enough to finish a task . . .	Use the goal-setting, break it down and take it on, or "A" list/"B" list exercises in Chapter 5.
If you have the desire to take a few risks . . .	Read the sections in this chapter on how to use the 24-hour rule and on getting feedback from others.

Clear and Unclear Definitions of Problems

Unclear definition	*Clear definition*
Paul thinks, "I'm lazy."	"I have not cleaned the apartment in several weeks."
Amanda says, "I'm broke."	"I may not have enough money to pay my phone bill this month because I had to get my car fixed."
Tommy thinks, "No one cares about me."	"My friends had a get-together this weekend, and no one invited me."
Raquel says, "I'm going to lose it if I get fired."	"It's possible that I will lose my job. I'm not sure what I will do for money if that happens or if I will be able to find another job."

Your definition of the problem should point you toward its solution. In the examples in the table, Paul needs to clean his apartment and Amanda needs to find money to pay the phone bill, ask the phone company to give her a break, or deal with having her phone service stopped. Tommy needs to make a decision to talk to his friends about being left out of the party or to get over it if it's not important enough to discuss with them. Raquel needs to find out if she will be fired soon and whether or not there is anything that can be done to stop it. If she is not sure what to do next, it may be time to begin looking for other job options or to ask others for advice or assistance.

To help you define and describe a problem clearly enough to solve it, ask yourself the following questions:

10 Questions to Define a Problem

1. What is the problem?
2. Is it something that happened in the past or something that still needs to be resolved?
3. Is it your problem or someone else's problem?
4. Is there anything you can do about it right now?

Go on to questions 5–10 only if it still needs to be resolved, it's your personal problem, and there is something you can do about it right now. If it's an old issue, not your problem, or there is nothing you can do about it now, use the exercises in Chapters 8 and 9 to work through your thoughts on the event.

  5. When is it most likely to occur?
  6. How often does the problem occur?
  7. If it does not get solved, what will happen?
  8. What is your biggest worry about this problem?
  9. If it were solved, how would things be different for you?
 10. What part of the problem needs to be solved first?

After you have given some thought to these 10 questions, fill in the blanks in Worksheet 10.1.

---

worksheet 10.1 | **Defining the Problem**

The problem is: _____

_____

The way it affects my life is: _____

_____

It upsets me because: _____

_____

It has to be resolved soon because: _____

_____

Paul's Worksheet 10.1

The problem is: *that my apartment is a mess.*

The way it affects my life is: *that it distracts me and makes me feel bad.*

It upsets me because: *I hate living in a disaster area.*

It has to be resolved soon because: *people might be coming over this weekend.*

Amanda's Worksheet 10.1

The problem is: _I don't have enough money._

The way it affects my life is: _that I can't pay all my bills._

It upsets me because: _this keeps happening to us. I hate living like this._

It has to be resolved soon because: _the bills are coming due._

Tommy's Worksheet 10.1

The problem is: _my friends blew me off._

The way it affects my life is: _I had nothing to do that night and I don't know why they did this._

It upsets me because: _these people are supposed to be my friends. I have lost friends before because of the problems I have had. I don't want to lose these._

It has to be resolved soon because: _it is going to keep bothering me until I know what happened._

Raquel's Worksheet 10.1

The problem is: _I might lose my job because I lost my temper with my boss._

The way it affects my life is: _I can't afford not to work. We need the money._

It upsets me because: _it was my fault. I shouldn't have overreacted. They are cutting jobs throughout the company. and I may have just hurt myself._

It has to be resolved soon because: _I am losing sleep over it and it is stressing me out._

• **Step 2: Find solutions.** The next step in problem solving is to put together a list of possible solutions. You can use Worksheet 10.2 to list your ideas. Try to come up with at least five possible solutions. One solution might be to change nothing and let the problem continue. Another might be to ask someone to solve it for you. While these may not be the best solutions, at least they are possibilities. Let yourself be as creative as possible in generating new solutions to your problem. Do not stop to evaluate each one as you think of it. Just make a list first and follow the steps for choosing the right one.

worksheet 10.2 | **Finding Solutions**

Possible solutions to my problem	
Order	**Ideas**

Raquel's Worksheet 10.2

Order	Ideas
	Apologize to my boss for jumping his case.
	Keep my mouth shut and wait to see what happens.
	Start looking for another job. Quit before I get fired.
	Ask my boss if he plans to fire me over what happened.
	Ask his secretary if she knows anything about his plan to fire me.

After you have filled in at least five possible solutions, cross off the ones that are least desirable or not very practical given your current situation. Think about the pros and cons of each of the remaining solutions and put them in order of preference. Place #1 in the narrow column on the left labeled "Order" next to your first choice, #2 next to your second choice, and so on. Solution #1 will usually be the first one you will try. If it looks like it's not going to work, go to solution #2 and so on.

Raquel has been fired twice before, and she does not want it to happen again. She knows she will be better off quitting before getting fired, but she doesn't want to jump the gun. She likes her job and the pay is good, so she would really rather not lose it. It would be better for her in the long run to do what she can to try to keep her job.

Raquel knows in her heart that she should probably apologize for what she said, but that's not easy for her to do. She is a proud woman and was not entirely wrong when she blew her stack at the boss. She doesn't know how to apologize for being rude without giving in on the issue.

She could also just ask her boss directly about his plans to fire her without apologizing. If it looked like he was heading in that direction, she could offer to resign instead. The problem with that idea is that she doesn't want to resign and she would not get unemployment benefits if she resigned.

After thinking it over, Raquel thought the wait-and-see method sounded like the easiest. She knew that sometimes she blew things out of proportion and jumped to conclusions about getting fired, so this could be another example of overreaction. Maybe her boss had forgiven her already for losing her cool. Maybe there was no problem. Raquel thought the best strategy would be to apologize to her boss for the way she handled their disagreement. That way she did not have to go back on what she said, just express regret for how she said it. Even if he was not about to fire her, offering an apology was probably the right thing to do. Her husband was much better at apologies than Raquel, so she would get him to help her write an e-mail to the boss. If she was going to get fired, she would find out soon enough. She would still have the option of offering to resign. It would be better for her and better for the company.

- **Step 3: Refine your plan.** Before you put your plan into action, think about
  - When you will try it.
  - Who will help you.
  - How you will know if it has worked.

Is it a solution you will try on your own, or do you need the cooperation of others? If other people are involved, talk over your ideas with them, get their suggestions, and make an agreement on when each of you will take action.

Raquel's Plan

➡ *When?* She will work with her husband tonight to write an apology note and send it tomorrow at work.

➡ *Who will help?* Her husband will help her write it. She will ask a friend at work to look it over and give her some feedback on how she thinks the boss will react.

➡ *How will she know if it has worked?* When her boss is mad, he ignores everyone; and when he is not mad, he is pretty friendly. If he makes conversation with her, she will know that he is not mad at her anymore. The lay-offs at work are scheduled for the next month. If she keeps her job, she will know that it has worked.

• **Step 4: Put your plan into action.** The next step is to try out your solution and see what happens. If the solution does not seem to work at first, make a decision to try it again or switch to solution #2 from your list. Sometimes you have to try the same solution more than once before it will work. If Raquel's apology note does not seem to make a difference, she may need to try again in person.

In other situations you may find that your first solution was not sufficient to address a problem. If that's the case, try another solution from your list.

If Raquel is uncertain how her note was received, she might ask the boss's secretary about it. Although she wishes she could just wait and see what happens to her job, Raquel knows that the wait will make her feel worse. If her first solution, the apology note, does not work, she will make an appointment and talk to the boss about her behavior and whether or not it will affect her job.

Learn from your experiences of success as well as failure. As you get to know yourself better—your motivations, your weaknesses, your abilities, and your needs—you will be able to choose solutions that best suit you.

Making Decisions

When you're making a choice between two options and one option stands out as better than the other, making a decision is easy. It gets more difficult when there are two or three less-than-perfect options and each has some definite advantages as well as some definite disadvantages.

Paul and his girlfriend have been together for 3 years. She has hinted around about marriage for the last 6 months. Angie is 2 years older than Paul and is ready to move on to the next stage of life. She wants to get married, buy a house, and have children. Angie loves Paul, but she thinks that he may be too immature to make this kind of commitment. She doesn't want to wait any longer, so she has asked Paul to marry her or let her go.

Paul loves Angie and doesn't want to lose her. She has stood by him as he has learned to control his illness and is tolerant of his "quirks." However, he is not sure he's ready for marriage. He has not accomplished his educational or financial goals and he may not be ready for the responsibilities of marriage, parenthood, and home ownership. Paul has to make a decision, and neither option, marriage or losing Angie, seemed like a good choice.

An even more complicated scenario arises when each choice has a clear advantage but the advantages are very different. Let's say you're choosing a place to live and you find two possibilities for about the same price. One has more space and the other has a better location. Which do you choose? Or what if you're choosing a college to go to and you're accepted by two, one where your closest friends are going and another that has a course of study you want to pursue. Which do you choose? If your thinking is clouded by emotion, overcrowded with racing thoughts, or slow and difficult to organize, you will have even more trouble making a decision. If you're like most people, you will put it off until you absolutely have to decide. Sometimes people will put off difficult decisions until the choice is made for them. For example, if Paul does not make a decision about marrying Angie, she will eventually leave him.

If you want to be more active in making decisions, you can follow the steps outlined in the next section. It will help you to sort out your options and choose the one that best meets your current needs. If you're not confident in your ability to reason through the choices, ask someone you trust for his or her opinion after you've completed the exercise.

- **Step 1**: List the choices you are weighing on the Decision-Making Worksheet (Worksheet 10.3). Work choices might include "I can change jobs," "I can remain at the existing job," and "I can apply for social security disability and stop working." If you're trying to make a decision to end a relationship, the choices might include "End it now," "Stick it out longer and hope it gets better," and "Tell my partner that I'm unhappy and ask if he [or she] is willing to work to make things better."
- **Step 2**: List the advantages and disadvantages of each choice. Some might overlap. For example, the advantages of staying at the same job (e.g., it is familiar and comfortable) might involve the same issue as the disadvantages of changing jobs (e.g., it would put you in a new and possibly scary situation). Overlap is OK. List every advantage and disadvantage you can think of. Ask a friend or a family member to help you think of other pros and cons to each choice.
- **Step 3**: Read through the lists and pick out one or two of the strongest advantages and disadvantages of each decision choice. Circle these items. If it would be easier to read, you can cross off the others on your list.
- **Step 4**: Look for common themes in the advantages and disadvantages you

listed. For example, if you're weighing the advantages and disadvantages of ending a relationship or staying with it, do you see *loneliness* versus *having someone to be with* as an issue? If so, it tells you that being with someone, not necessarily the person you are with now, is important to you. If you see stress reduction showing up as an advantage of making a change in jobs as well as a disadvantage of staying in your current job, then you know that your stress level is an important issue in your decisions. If you are trying to decide whether or not to change doctors, you might find the theme of familiarity and hating change in your advantages and disadvantages.

Examine the main advantages and disadvantages that you circled in Step 3 and try to pick out the main themes. List them on the Decision-Making Worksheet under "Themes."

- **Step 5:** To the right of each, rank-order the themes/issues according to their importance in making your decision. Make #1 the most important theme, #2 the second most important theme, and so on.

- **Step 6:** Once you have picked out the most important themes that will guide your decision making on a given problem and have arranged them in order of importance, it's time to match the themes to each of the decision options. This means going back to your original list of decision choices and picking out the ones that best match each theme. For example, if loneliness was the most important theme in making a decision about a relationship, pick the decision choice from your list of possible options that would be best for reducing your loneliness. If the second theme you identified was concern about money, go back to the list of decision choices and pick the one that best addresses your concern about money. To help you keep track, write the decision choice number from the Decision-Making Worksheet next to each theme that it matches.

- **Step 7:** Now that you have a list of themes and the decision choices that best match each theme, you can compare the items and choose the decision that addresses your issues best. You will know which it is by the number of themes each decision choice addresses. So if the decision choice you labeled #1 on the Decision-Making Worksheet does a good job of addressing each of the themes you identified, it's probably the best choice. If another decision choice addressed only one of your themes, and it was not the most important theme, it's probably not a good choice. The best options are those decision choices that address the most themes or issues or that at least address the most important themes.

Paul decided to share this worksheet with Angie and ask her to do the same thing. If she was willing to wait, he was willing to commit to marriage. He needed time to prepare himself. This included finishing school. If he took more classes and worked fewer hours, he could finish in three more semesters. While he was finishing his degree he would work with his therapist on his emotional readiness and ask Angie to join them for some of their sessions. If Angie was not willing to wait, there was nothing he could do.

Decision-Making Worksheet

Possible options	Advantages	Disadvantages
Option 1:		
Option 2:		
Option 3:		

Themes	Order of importance	Best options

From *The Bipolar Workbook* by Monica Ramirez Basco. Copyright 2006 by The Guilford Press. Permission to photocopy this form is granted to purchasers of this book for personal use only (see copyright page for details).

Paul's Worksheet 10.3

Possible options	Advantages	Disadvantages
Option 1: Marry Angie	I get to keep her forever. She'll be happy and won't leave me. We can start working on building the lives we want.	I'm too young. I'll give up my independence. I won't have my parents to back me up financially. Marriage means more debt. Being together 24/7.
Option 2: Break up with Angie	I will be able to finish my education without having to worry about money. I can date other people. I can hang out with my friends whenever I want. I don't have to burden Angie with my mood swings.	I will miss her terribly. I will never find anyone like her again. No one else will want to deal with my moodiness. I have to give up my dream of life and children with her. I will get severely depressed.
Option 3: Find a way to postpone marriage	I can keep Angie. I can take time to finish school and save some money. I can get ready to be a husband.	Angie says that she will not wait. If I postpone it too long, she will give up on me. She will start to hate me for making her put off her plans.

Themes	Order of importance	Best options
Losing Angie	1	1
Money	3	2, ③
Having someone who can understand me	2	1, ③
Being emotionally ready	4	2, ③

Here is another example.

Tommy had to move back in with his parents after his last hospitalization. He had been living with them for nine months and thought he was ready to be on his own. His parents had paid for his apartments in the past, but he had always had to move back home either because he got evicted for excessive noise or for not keeping the place clean or because he was too ill to live on his own. Tommy's parents were not willing to go through that again, so they told him that if he wanted to live on his own he would have to pay for his own apartment. Tommy could not decide what to do, so he filled out Worksheet 10.3 to help him sort through the issues. The choices he was considering were moving out on his own, getting a roommate, and continuing to stay with his parents for a while.

After he had worked through the exercise, it became clear to Tommy that his best option would be to find a roommate and move out on his own. This choice addressed the issues or themes he had identified better than the other two options. He had a friend who lived in a one-bedroom apartment in the same city and was willing to rent a bigger apartment with Tommy and share expenses.

Tommy's Worksheet 10.3

Possible options	Advantages	Disadvantages
Option 1: Move out on my own	Independence No one to stress me Peace and quiet	Costs more money Loneliness Not sure I can handle it
Option 2: Get a roommate	Share expenses Might be fun Don't have to be alone	We might not get along. Limits my privacy We might have different habits.
Option 3: Live with my mom & dad	Save money for the future Have my own room Never lonely	No privacy Mom tells me what to do. Can't have people over

Themes	Order of importance	Best options
Independence, being on my own, and privacy	2	1, 2
Money	1	2, 3
Loneliness versus having someone around to talk to	3	2, 3

Getting Feedback from Others

You may not want to admit it, but sometimes other people who know you are right about what you should or should not do. They may be able to help you sort through your many ideas, decisions, choices, urges, and worries. Other people can be a resource if you let them. They may not always be right, but they can offer ideas that are different than yours and therefore challenge you to consider other possibilities.

When you are manic or hypomanic, you may have a lot more thoughts to sort through than usual. You also run the risk of making mistakes in logic and making poor choices because you've overlooked important facts. Most people regret making bad decisions when they are manic and want to learn methods for stopping themselves the next time before they act. The kinds of ideas that should alert you to be cautious are urges to make big changes in your life, to do something impulsive that would shock or surprise others, and to take risks that you would not normally take. When these ideas run through your mind, one strategy for protecting yourself is to tell someone about it. Even if you don't want the person's opinion or couldn't care less about his or her reaction, hearing yourself say the idea out loud can be enough to make you think it through before you act impulsively and regret it later.

Some people who have bipolar disorder don't feel comfortable verbalizing their impulsive thoughts because it makes other people overreact, become suspicious, watch them too closely, or behave in other negative ways toward them. These are valid concerns. No one wants to have a great idea shot down. On the other hand, to keep yourself out of trouble, you may need someone to help you apply the brakes. Identify a person in your world that you can talk to about your ideas that others might find outrageous. Make sure it's someone who knows that just because you're thinking about taking risks doesn't mean you will actually do it. A therapist or psychiatrist can be that person, but it may be more practical to choose a family member, a friend, or someone else you know who has bipolar disorder and deals with similar thoughts from time to time. If you share your idea and get a negative reaction, apply the 24-hour rule.

➡ *What's Next?*

Congratulations! You've worked through the first three steps in the CBT approach to the treatment of bipolar disorder. If you've done the exercises in the workbook, you've learned to see symptoms coming, take precautions to keep them from returning, and reduce your symptoms when they occur. Now it's time to take the fourth and final step: check your progress. The next chapter will help you put the pieces of the program together by summarizing the overall strategy. You will have a chance to plan out your long-term strategy for using the methods in this workbook.

If you've read through the workbook without doing the exercises, now is the time to go back and work through the ones that apply to you. Remember that the boxes at the beginning of each chapter give you a brief summary of the chapter's content. They will help you pick and choose which chapters and exercises to complete. You don't have to complete all the exercises at one sitting. It's probably best to use the workbook in an ongoing way as you experience the mood swings and symptoms that have been covered throughout the book. If you're not sure where to start, read the next chapter. A summary of the basic steps for taking control of your illness is provided. Reacquaint yourself with the basic procedures and pick a place to start the program.

Step 4

Check Your Progress

chapter eleven

Making Changes for the Better

> *In this chapter you will:*
> ✓ Review the aims of this workbook.
> ✓ Check your progress.
> ✓ Set goals for continued improvement.
> ✓ Read about common obstacles to achieving your treatment goals.

The goal of this workbook is to teach you something about the management of bipolar disorder. To check how much progress you've made in learning the principles covered, retake the test from the beginning of the book (Worksheet 11.1) and see if your knowledge of bipolar disorder has improved.

Reexamining the Big Picture

The overall goal of this workbook has been to teach you methods:

- to prevent recurrences of depression and mania
- to know when symptoms are returning
- to take action to control symptoms before they become full episodes of depression and mania, and
- to correct and control the thinking problems, activity changes, and emotional upsets caused by the illness

The outline on pages 230–232, which you saw in Chapter 1, too, summarizes the steps you can take to make changes for the better. The interventions throughout the workbook are geared toward helping you in four ways—to see it coming, take precautions, reduce your symptoms, and check your progress.

| **Knowledge Test**

Test Your Knowledge of Bipolar Disorder

Circle *true* or *false*. The correct answers are on pages viii–x.

True or False   1. Bipolar disorder can cause both depression and mania.

True or False   2. You can be depressed and manic at the same time.

True or False   3. Medications are necessary to control the symptoms of bipolar disorder.

True or False   4. All you need to do to stay well is take your medication every day.

True or False   5. There is nothing you can do to stop depression or mania once it starts.

True or False   6. Sleep loss can trigger a manic episode.

True or False   7. To cope with bipolar disorder, you have to give up the exciting parts of life.

True or False   8. Having the illness usually means giving up your career goals.

True or False   9. You can handle this illness on your own. You don't need help.

True or False   10. You don't have bipolar disorder. The doctors are wrong.

Step 1: See It Coming

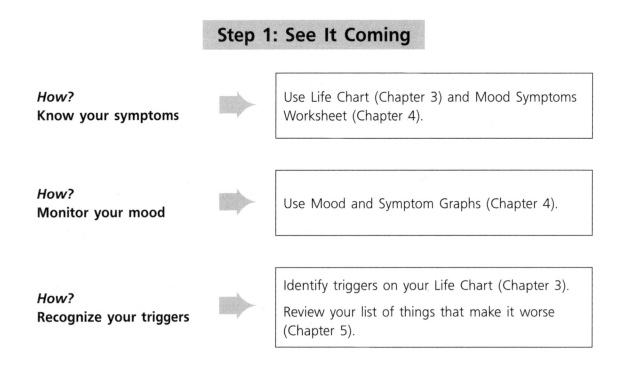

How?
Know your symptoms ➡ Use Life Chart (Chapter 3) and Mood Symptoms Worksheet (Chapter 4).

How?
Monitor your mood ➡ Use Mood and Symptom Graphs (Chapter 4).

How?
Recognize your triggers ➡ Identify triggers on your Life Chart (Chapter 3).

Review your list of things that make it worse (Chapter 5).

Step 2: Take Precautions

How?
Don't make it worse ➔ Learn to get enough sleep (Chapter 5).

Stick with medications (Chapter 6).

Avoid symptom triggers (Chapters 5 and 6).

How?
Add positives ➔ Learn to strengthen relationships (Chapters 5 and 8).

Set personal goals (Chapter 6).

Work toward adjustment to the illness (Chapter 7).

Develop healthy habits (Chapter 5).

How?
Decrease negatives ➔ Solve problems (Chapters 5 and 8).

Control worry and rumination (Chapter 5).

Avoid overstimulation (Chapters 5 and 9).

Step 3: Reduce Your Symptoms

How?
Stop inactivity ➔ Use Activity Schedule.

Break it down and take it on, and use "A" list/"B" list (Chapter 5).

How?
Change your thinking ➔ Use the *catch it, control it, correct it* methods (Chapters 8 and 9).

How?
Reverse mental meltdown ➔ Use the *slow it, focus it, structure it* methods (Chapter 10).

How?
Reduce hyperactivity ➔ Control overstimulation.

Keep desire for change in check.

Set limits on activity with goal setting.

Get some sleep (Chapter 5).

Step 4: Check Your Progress

How?
Monitor your mood and symptom changes

→

Use Mood Graphs (Chapter 4).

Use Mood Symptoms Worksheet (Chapter 4).

Get feedback from others (Chapter 9).

Checking Your Progress

The exercises provided throughout the workbook have encouraged you to be specific about your goals and your plans. Now that you've read through the various methods for controlling your symptoms of depression and mania, make a few notes on Worksheet 11.2 about the steps you have already taken or plan to take to accomplish each of these aims.

The goals emphasized throughout this workbook are:

- To **know yourself**, your vulnerabilities, your strengths, and your symptoms well
- To **practice** and strengthen the skills for managing your illness that have been described in this workbook
- To **learn from each episode** of illness you experience so that you know what to watch for next time
- To **work toward acceptance** of having bipolar disorder so that you can move forward, do everything you can to stay well, and get on with your life
- To **avoid risks** of relapse
- To **find a medication** regimen you feel comfortable enough to follow

Monitoring Your Mood

The methods you learned in Chapter 4 for recognizing symptoms of depression and mania and for monitoring daily mood changes can help you keep check on your progress. If you were rating yourself regularly on a Mood Graph (see Worksheet 11.3), what you would hope to see is a steady improvement in your mood over time and then more stability in your mood. That means that if you rated your mood each day and connected the dots on the graph, you would see a line through the middle with fluctuations between –1 and +1 most of the time. When your mood dropped toward depression or climbed toward mania, you would hope to see those changes return to normal within a few days. And if you use the new tools you have learned

| **My Plans for Managing My Bipolar Disorder**

Ways I have gotten to know my vulnerabilities, my strengths, and my symptoms better. My plan for learning more about myself and my illness.

My thoughts on how to practice and strengthen my skills for managing my illness that have been described in this workbook.

How I might learn from each episode of illness I experience so that I know what to watch for next time.

What I need to do to work toward acceptance of having bipolar disorder so that I can move forward, do everything I can to stay well, and get on with my life.

Things I know I can do to avoid the risk of relapse.

How I will find a medication regimen I feel comfortable enough to follow.

in this workbook as often as possible, you should have fewer and fewer days with ratings above +2 or below −2.

If you decide not to keep Mood Graphs on a daily basis, you can use them periodically to check on how you're doing. For example, if you know you tend to get depressed in the winter and manic during the spring, you might start keeping a mood graph just before those seasons begin. If you see that your graph is moving toward more symptoms, use the methods you've learned to stop their progression and contact your doctor when you see that the daily ratings are not improving or that the symptoms are becoming more difficult to manage on your own. When the season is over, keep a Mood Graph for another week or two to be certain that your mood is remaining stable.

Adjustment and Acceptance

If you've struggled with acceptance of having bipolar disorder, your efforts throughout this workbook may have helped you progress through the stages of adjustment. Review the thoughts and behaviors associated with each stage of adjustment (Worksheet 11.4) to see if you can recognize where you are today. Compare your answers to those you marked on Worksheet 7.1 in Chapter 7.

You Don't Have to Do It Alone

Workbooks like this one can make interventions seem easy, but they may be more difficult when you try to put them into action. It can be very helpful to have a therapist who is familiar with bipolar disorder work with you. Not all therapists have had experience with this particular illness, so you will want to ask them about their comfort with treating bipolar disorder before you get started.

The **Depression and Bipolar Support Alliance** is a national organization committed to education and support of people who have mood disorders such as depression and bipolar disorders. They have chapters all over the country that provide educational lectures by professionals, group discussions for people who suffer from these illnesses, discussion groups for family members, and a library of educational materials and books. To find a DBSA group in your area, you can go to the organization's website at DBSAlliance.org. There you will find information about the organization and a map for locating a DBSA group in your area.

Obstacles to Achieving Your Treatment Goals

Changing the course of your illness is a tall order. Most people question their ability to create a life with fewer periods of depression and mania. Because it is a lifelong

| **Mood Graph**

Week of:								
	Plan	**Su**	**M**	**T**	**W**	**Th**	**F**	**Sa**
Manic								
+5 Not sleeping, psychotic	*Go to the hospital*	•	•	•	•	•	•	•
+4 Manic, poor judgment		•	•	•	•	•	•	•
+3 Hypomanic	*Call the doctor*	•	•	•	•	•	•	•
+2 Hyper	*Take action*	•	•	•	•	•	•	•
+1 Happy, up	*Watch closely*	•	•	•	•	•	•	•
0 Normal		•	•	•	•	•	•	•
−1 Low, down	*Watch closely*	•	•	•	•	•	•	•
−2 Sad	*Take action*	•	•	•	•	•	•	•
−3 Depressed	*Call the doctor*	•	•	•	•	•	•	•
−4 Immobilized		•	•	•	•	•	•	•
−5 Suicidal	*Go to the hospital*	•	•	•	•	•	•	•
Depressed								

What caused the mood shift?

| worksheet 11.4 | **Stages of Adjustment to Bipolar Disorder** |

Stage	Automatic thoughts	Actions
Denial	• I don't have it. The doctor made a mistake. • It must be because I've been drinking too much. • The diagnosis is wrong.	• Getting a second opinion. • Looking for other explanations for symptoms. • Ignoring treatment recommendations.
Anger	• It's not fair that I have this illness. • I can't deal with this right now. • Why me? What did I do to deserve this?	• Refusing to listen to advice. • Refusing to discuss the illness. • Losing temper with health care providers, pharmacies, or anyone else associated with treatment.
Bargaining	• I'll clean up my act. • I'll stop drinking, start waking up on time, start exercising, get a better job, and it will be OK. • I'll try natural remedies. I don't really need medicine.	• Adjusting doses on your own. • Changing the timing of doses. • Trading active drugs for "natural remedies." • Staying up late to avoid taking sleeping medications. • Drinking alcohol to reduce anxiety.
Depression	• I'll never have a normal life. • No one will want me. • I hate myself.	• Self-destructive behaviors. • Avoidance of doctors, magazine articles, or anything else that reminds you of the illness. • Withdrawal from others.
Acceptance	• I can work my way through this. • It's not the end of the world. • I don't have to give up everything just because I have to take medication.	• Adherence with treatment. • Open discussion of treatment options with clinicians before discontinuing medications.

battle, it's easy to lose steam and think about giving up along the way. Here are some examples of common thoughts people have about controlling their symptoms of bipolar disorder, along with some advice for keeping these thoughts from interfering with your goals.

"I don't want to take precautions."

If taking precautions by keeping a more consistent sleep schedule, monitoring your symptoms, and limiting overstimulation sounds like too much restriction on your lifestyle, you may not want to do it. You certainly have the right to do as you please, take the risks you want, and deal with any consequences that may follow. It's your decision to follow or not follow the guidelines in this workbook, to take the advice of your therapist, or to take medication the way your doctor tells you to. If you live alone and do not have responsibilities to others, you will be the only one to suffer the costs of not taking precautions. It may not be a big deal. But if other people depend on you and a return of your depression or mania will affect their lives, your decision should probably take them into consideration.

Be sure not to view taking precautions in an all-or-nothing way. It's not a matter of total restriction versus total freedom. You may be able to make some changes in your routine to better suit your illness or try to take precautions as often as possible, knowing there will be times when your lifestyle will not allow it. Also consider the possibility that you may not be ready to make the kind of changes in your routine that are being recommended by the workbook, your family, or your health care providers. That doesn't mean you won't be more ready next month or next year or the next time you have symptoms. Taking care of yourself will always be a good idea no matter when you start taking the right action. If you know you can't do it right now, put this book back on your shelf and look it over again later. Life circumstances can change quickly and create new opportunities for you to take control of your symptoms.

"It's not going to help."

This idea is a good example of jumping to conclusions. If you believe that an exercise will not help, then you will skip it. Avoiding the activity will not help you feel any better either. Instead of trusting your feelings, try to be objective. Test your theory that it isn't going to help by giving it a try. You may be right and will have to try a different strategy, or you may be wrong and find that it helps.

"I can't do it."

If you are a black-and-white thinker like Amanda, and the exercise you're trying doesn't make you feel better right away, you may give up on it too easily. Progress may be noticeable but small at first. For example, if you're trying to combat the negative thought "I'm stupid," after evaluating the evidence you may be partially but not completely convinced that you were wrong about yourself. If you have held on to a negative view of yourself for a long time, it will take some work to convince yourself otherwise. You have to retrain your thought process by continually practicing methods for evaluating and correcting your overly negative ideas. With practice, change can become permanent. So if you find yourself thinking "I can't do it," and feeling frustrated, take a break and then try again, because giving up too soon will only reinforce your negative thoughts.

"The medicine is working now, so I don't have to try."

Even when medication works well, a number of things can cause you to have a recurrence of depression or mania. For example, using alcohol or street drugs can induce symptoms. Sleep loss over several days can make mania return. Suffering a major loss or crisis in your life can cause depression to return. Even the changing of the seasons can bring symptoms back. A major medical illness, a car accident, or giving birth can all cause you to have a relapse, even if you're taking medication for bipolar disorder. There may be nothing you can do to prevent accidents or injuries, but you can take control over your own actions that can put you at risk for relapse. Medications are essential for treatment, but they are not 100% effective. How you take them, when you take them, how you manage your lifestyle, and how you react when symptoms return are all ways in which you have control over the course of your illness.

"The symptoms came back anyway."

Many people will master the techniques in this workbook but find that their symptoms return anyway. Because bipolar disorder is a recurring illness, you should count on there being times when your symptoms return. There are a few lucky people who find exactly the right medication, take it religiously, and never have mania or depression again. Unfortunately, they are not in the majority. The goal of managing bipolar disorder is to decrease the number of episodes of depression and mania as much possible, eliminate the milder symptoms that can continue between episodes, and, if a relapse does occur, catch and contain it as quickly as possible. This way you will spend more time feeling well and less time feeling ill as you learn more and more about controlling the illness.

"It's not worth it. I give up."

The statement "It's not worth it " suggests that you have weighed the value of trying to control your bipolar disorder against the gains that come with feeling well and have decided that the costs of trying outweigh the benefits of well-being. Therefore, the effort is not worth the benefits you receive. This could be considered a thinking error of magnification of the negative and minimization of the positive, or it could be true. If you are not getting what you need out of medication treatment or psychotherapy, rather than giving it up, perhaps you should consider the possibility that it's time for a change. People change medications, doctors, and therapists all the time until they find one worth the cost and effort. If your treatment were better matched to your illness, perhaps it would be worth it to you.

"I'm tired of trying."

Depression, medication side effects, running out of money, and pressure from other people can all make you want to give up on treatment. The low energy, loss of motivation, mental slowness, and hopelessness that are brought about by depression can also convince you that you would be better off if you didn't take medicine, stopped going to doctors, and gave up on the endless struggle to control your illness. The effort it takes to manage your illness can leave you mentally and emotionally exhausted at times. To cope with these feelings, some people take breaks from trying to control their illness. For a few days they feel a sense of freedom, but unfortunately, the symptoms return.

Wanting to give up because you're tired of trying is a normal feeling. People feel that way when they are tired of their jobs, tired of school, tired of taking care of small children, tired of trying to get out of debt, and tired of trying to find the right partner. If you're facing these kinds of life struggles along with trying to control your illness, you have the right to be especially exhausted. Life can be very hard. To cope with these times, you have to add positives to your life to balance out all the negatives. If you have some good things to look forward to, people who give you pleasure or make you smile, reasons to rush home after a long day at work, these things will help you hang in there and put out the effort to be at your best. If you lack positives in your life, it's time to add them. A few examples are provided in Chapter 5, but use your imagination to make your life worth the effort it takes to stay well.

Planning Ahead to Accomplish Your Goals

In Chapter 6, "Getting the Most Out of Medication," behavioral contracts were introduced as a way of planning ahead for obstacles that might interfere with your achieving your treatment goals. Take a moment and think about what could keep you from achieving the goals of this workbook and write them on Worksheet 11.5.

If you use the methods in this workbook, you'll find that with practice you will be able to:

- See it coming,
- Take precautions,
- Reduce your symptoms, and
- Check your progress.

Remember that each time you experience depression, mania, hypomania, or mixed states, you have an opportunity to put your new tools to the test, evaluate their precision, and refine them for times to come.

▶ What's Next?

Now that you've learned the tools for controlling your symptoms of bipolar disorder, it's time to put them into practice. Controlling the symptoms of bipolar disorder is an ongoing process. This workbook was written to help you through that process. Refer back to the guidelines and exercises as you encounter symptoms or problems along the way. Even when times are good and you are feeling fine, review the strategies for staying well and for managing your lifestyle.

Share your work with your doctor or therapist so that he or she will know what you're doing to manage your illness. Find a way to remind yourself from time to time to check on your symptoms and make the adjustments you've learned to keep them under control.

If you hit a rough spot and depression or mania returns, do your part to pull yourself together. Learn from the experience by analyzing what occurred that might have made you vulnerable to relapse. Each time you have symptoms and get them under control, you learn more about how to prevent them the next time.

| **Overcoming Obstacles to Improvement**

Goal: Prevent recurrences of depression and mania

Potential obstacles to achieving this goal:

What I can do to overcome these obstacles:

Goal: Learn when my symptoms are returning

Potential obstacles to achieving this goal:

What I can do to overcome these obstacles:

(cont.)

Goal: Take action to control symptoms before they become full episodes of depression and mania

Potential obstacles to achieving this goal:

What I can do to overcome these obstacles:

Goal: Correct and control the thinking problems, activity changes, and emotional upsets caused by the illness

Potential obstacles to achieving this goal:

What I can do to overcome these obstacles:

Resources

Books

General Information on Bipolar and Other Mood Disorders

An Unquiet Mind: A Memoir of Moods and Madness by Kay R. Jamison. New York: Random House, 1995.

The Bipolar Disorder Survival Guide: What You and Your Family Need to Know by David J. Miklowitz. New York: Guilford Press, 2002.

Exuberance: The Passion for Life by Kay R. Jamison. New York: Knopf, 2004.

Getting Your Life Back: A Complete Guide to Recovery from Depression by Jesse H. Wright and Monica Ramirez Basco. New York: Touchstone Books, 2003.

The Hypomanic Edge: The Link between (a Little) Craziness and (a Lot of) Success in America by J. D. Gartner. New York: Simon & Schuster, 2005.

New Hope for People with Bipolar Disorder by Jan Fawcett, Bernard Golden, and Nancy Rosenfeld. Roseville, CA: Prima Publishing, 2000.

Surviving Manic Depression: A Manual on Bipolar Disorder for Patients, Families, and Providers. New York: Basic Books, 2002.

Why Am I Up and Why Am I Down: Understanding Bipolar Disorder by Roger Granet and Elizabeth Ferber. New York: Dell Publications, 1999.

For Family and Friends

Loving Someone with Bipolar Disorder: Understanding and Helping Your Partner by Julie A. Fast and John D. Preston. Oakland, CA: New Harbinger Publications, Inc., 2004.

Raising a Moody Child: How to Cope with Depression and Bipolar Disorder by Mary A. Fristad and Jill S. Goldberg-Arnold. New York: Guilford Press, 2004.

For Professionals

*The Bipolar Child: The Definitive and Reassuring Guide to Childhood's Most Misunder-
stood Disorder, Revised and Expanded Edition* by Demitri Papolos and Janice Papolos.
New York: Broadway Books, 2002.

Cognitive-Behavioral Therapy for Bipolar Disorder, Second edition by Monica Ramirez
Basco and A. John Rush. New York: Guilford Press, 2005.

Structured Group Therapy for Bipolar Disorder: The Life Goals Program, Second Edition
by Mark S. Bauer and Linda McBride. New York: Springer Publishing Co., 2003.

Treating Bipolar Disorder: A Clinician's Guide to Interpersonal and Social Rhythm Therapy
by Ellen Frank. New York: Guilford Press, 2005.

Advocacy and Support Groups for Bipolar Disorder

Depression and Bipolar Support Alliance
(800) 826-3632
www.dbsalliance.org

A national nonprofit organization dedicated to improving the lives of people with mood disorders.

Child & Adolescent Bipolar Foundation
(847) 256-8525
www.bpkids.org

A parent-led, not-for-profit organization that supports and advocates on behalf of families
raising children diagnosed with or at risk for early-onset bipolar disorder.

National Alliance for the Mentally Ill
(800) 950-NAMI
www.nami.org

A national nonprofit advocacy group to help people with mental illness; their website includes information specific to bipolar disorder and information on state and local affiliates.

Step Up for BP Kids
(866) 992-KIDS
www.stepup4bpkids.org

A nonprofit foundation benefiting children and adolescents with early-onset bipolar disorder.

Additional Online Resources for Bipolar Disorder

Yahoo Health Depression Center
http://health.yahoo.com/centers/depression/0926

National Institute of Mental Health Booklet on Bipolar Disorder
www.nimh.nih.gov/publicat/bipolar.cfm

McMan's Depression and Bipolar Web
www.mcmanweb.com

Bipolar Significant Others
www.bpso.org

Find the Light Mental Health Support Group
www.findthelight.net/bipolar/mania.htm

Mayo Clinic Mental Health Center Information on Bipolar Disorder
www.mayoclinic.com/invoke.cfm?id=ds00356

Guide to Bipolar Disorder
www.bipolarhome.org

Bipolar World
www.bipolarworld.net

Index

About the Author

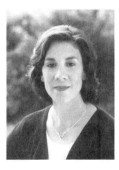

Monica Ramirez Basco, PhD, is a clinical psychologist, author, lecturer, and Clinical Associate Professor of Psychology at the University of Texas Southwestern Medical Center at Dallas. She is an internationally recognized expert in cognitive-behavioral therapy and a founding fellow of the Academy of Cognitive Therapy. Dr. Basco is the author of *Never Good Enough: How to Use Perfectionism to Your Advantage without Letting It Ruin Your Life* and coauthor of *Getting Your Life Back: The Complete Guide to Recovery from Depression* and *Cognitive-Behavioral Therapy for Bipolar Disorder* (2nd ed.). She has written numerous magazine articles and has appeared on national television programs, including *Today* and *The Oprah Winfrey Show.*